The Bean Fanatic's Mediterranean Cookbook

How to Cook Complete Meals with Beans and Grains Like A True Mediterranean

By
Delia Bell

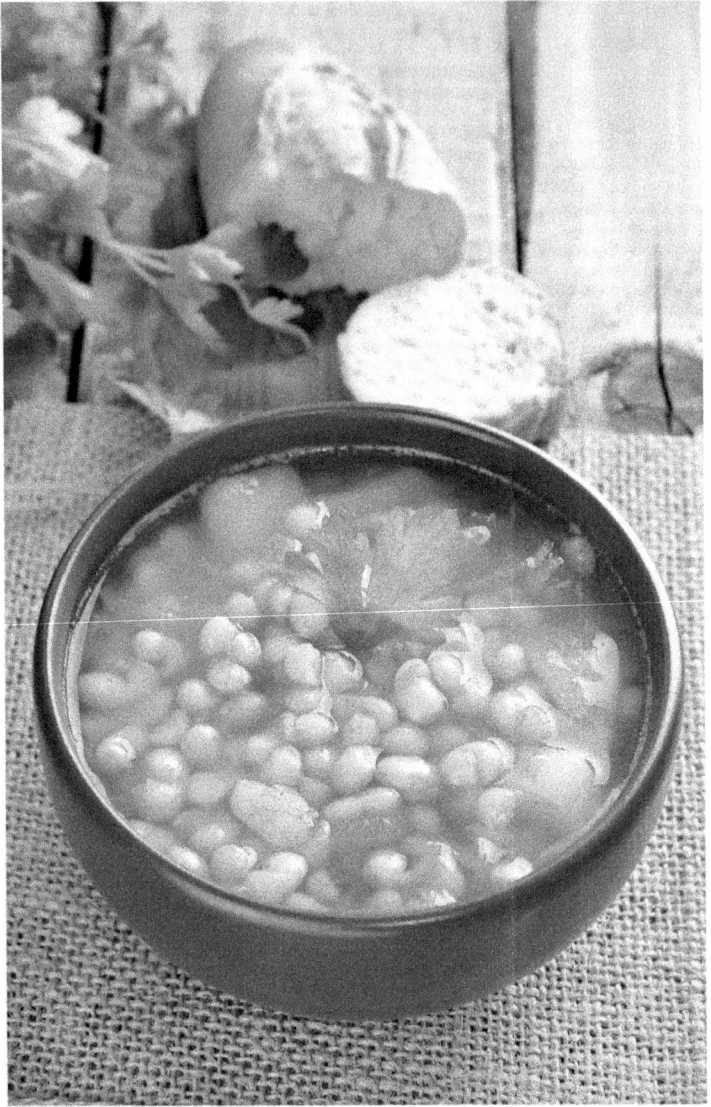

Table of Contents

INTRODUCTION   7

What is the Mediterranean Diet?   7

Cucumber Olive Rice   13

Chorizo-kidney Beans Quinoa Pilaf   15

Belly-filling Cajun Rice & Chicken   17

Chicken And White Bean   18

Quinoa & Black Bean Stuffed Sweet Potatoes   20

Feta, Eggplant And Sausage Penne   22

Bell Peppers 'n Tomato-chickpea Rice   23

Lip Smacking Chicken Tetrazzini   25

Spaghetti In Lemon Avocado White Sauce   26

Kidney Beans And Beet Salad   29

Filling Macaroni Soup   30

Simple Penne Antipasto   33

Squash And Eggplant Casserole   34

Blue Cheese And Grains Salad   37

Creamy Artichoke Lasagna   40

Brown Rice Pilaf With Butternut Squash   43

Cranberry And Roasted Squash Delight   45

Spanish Rice Casserole With Cheesy Beef   47

Kidney Bean And Parsley-lemon Salad   49

Italian White Bean Soup   51

Mexican Quinoa Bake   53

Citrus Quinoa & Chickpea Salad   54

Chickpea Salad Moroccan Style   56

Garlicky Peas And Clams On Veggie Spiral   57

Leek, Bacon And Pea Risotto   60

Chickpea Fried Eggplant Salad   62

Turkey And Quinoa Stuffed Peppers	65
Pastitsio An Italian Dish	67
Rice And Chickpea Stew	70
Mediterranean Diet Pasta With Mussels	72
Brussels Sprouts 'n White Bean Medley	75
Sun-dried Tomatoes And Chickpeas	76
Puttanesca Style Bucatini	78
Garlic Avocado-pesto And Zucchini Pasta	79
Mushroom Chickpea Marsala	81
Creamy Alfredo Fettuccine	82
Chickpea-crouton Kale Caesar Salad	84
Lemon Asparagus Risotto	85
Seafood Paella With Couscous	88
Greek Farro Salad	90
Exotic Chickpea Tagine	93
Amazingly Good Parsley Tabbouleh	95
Zucchini And Brown Rice	97
Perfect Herb Rice	98
Fiber Packed Chicken Rice	99
Baked Parmesan And Eggplant Pasta	100
Greek Couscous Salad And Herbed Lamb Chops	103
Fresh Herbs And Clams Linguine	105
Garbanzo And Lentil Soup	106
Pasta And Tuna Salad	108
Quinoa Buffalo Bites	109
Feta On Tomato-black Bean	110

INTRODUCTION

What is the Mediterranean Diet?

The Mediterranean diet is based on the diets of traditional eating habits from the 1960s of people from countries that surround the Mediterranean Sea, such as Greece, Italy, and Spain, and it encourages the consumption of fresh, seasonal, and local foods. The Mediterranean diet has become popular because individuals show low rates of heart disease, chronic disease, and obesity. The Mediterranean diet profile focuses on whole grains, good fats (fish, olive oil, nuts etc.), vegetables, fruits, fish, and very low consumption of any non-fish meat. Along with food, the Mediterranean diet emphasizes the need to spend time eating with family and physical activity. The Mediterranean diet is not a single prescribed diet, but rather a general food-based eating pattern, which is marked by local and cultural differences throughout the Mediterranean region.

The diet is generally characterized by a high intake of plant-based foods (e.g. fresh fruit and vegetables, nuts, and cereals) and olive oil, a moderate intake of fish and poultry, and low intakes of dairy products (mostly yoghurt and cheese), red and processed meats, and sweets. Wine is typically consumed in moderation and, normally, with a meal. A strong focus is placed on social and cultural aspects, such as communal mealtimes, resting after eating, and regular physical activity. Nowadays, however, the diet is no longer followed as widely as it was 30-50 years ago, as the diets of people living in these regions are becoming more 'Westernized' and higher in energy dense foods.

Benefits

The Mediterranean diet is not a weight loss, but increasing fiber intake and cutting out red meat, animal fats, and processed food may lead to weight loss. People who follow the diet may also have a lower risk of various diseases.

Heart health

In the 1950s,an American scientist, found that people living in the poorer areas of southern Italy had a lower risk of heart disease and death than those in wealthier parts of New York. Dr. Keys attributed this to diet. Since then, many studies have indicated that following a Mediterranean diet can help the body maintain healthy cholesterol levels and reduce the risk of high blood pressure and cardiovascular disease. The overall pattern of the Mediterranean diet is similar to their own dietary recommendations. A high proportion of calories on the diet come from fat, which can increase the risk of obesity. However, they also note that this fat is mainly unsaturated, which makes it a more healthful option than that from the typical American diet.

Protection from disease

The Mediterranean diet focuses on plant-based foods, and these are good sources of antioxidants.

The Mediterranean diet might offer protection from various cancers, and especially colorectal cancer. The reduction in risk may stem from the high intake of fruits, vegetables, and whole grains. By sticking to Mediterranean meals, people's levels of blood glucose and fats had decreased. During this time, there was also a lower incidence of stroke.

Diabetes

The Mediterranean diet may help prevent type 2 diabetes and improve markers of diabetes in people who already have the condition. Various other studies have concluded that following the Mediterranean diet can reduce the risk of type 2 diabetes and cardiovascular disease, which often occur together.

Food to eat

There is no single definition of the Mediterranean diet, but one group of scientists used the following as their 2015 basis of research.

Vegetables: Include 3 to 9 servings a day.

Fresh fruit: Up to 2 servings a day.

Cereals: Mostly whole grain from 1 to 13 servings a day.

Oil: Up to 8 servings of extra virgin (cold pressed) olive oil a day.

Fat — mostly unsaturated — made up 37% of the total calories. Unsaturated fat comes from plant sources, such as olives and avocado. The Mediterranean diet also provided 33 grams (g) of fiber a day. The baseline diet for this study provided around

2,200 calories a day. Typical ingredients. Here are some examples of ingredients that people often include in the Mediterranean diet.

Vegetables: Tomatoes, peppers, onions, eggplant, zucchini, cucumber, leafy green vegetables, plus others.

Fruits: Melon, apples, apricots, peaches, oranges, and lemons, and so on.

Legumes: Beans, lentils, and chickpeas.

Nuts and seeds: Almonds, walnuts, sunflower seeds, and cashews.

Unsaturated fat: Olive oil, sunflower oil, olives, and avocados.

Dairy products: Cheese and yogurt are the main dairy foods.

Cereals: These are mostly whole grain and include wheat and rice with bread accompanying many meals.

Fish: Sardines and other oily fish, as well as oysters and other shellfish. Poultry: Chicken or turkey.

Eggs: Chicken, quail, and duck eggs.

Drinks: A person can drink red wine in moderation.

The Mediterranean diet does not include strong liquor or carbonated and sweetened drinks. According to one definition, the diet limits red meat and sweets to less than 2 servings per week.

Food to avoid

Here's a list of foods you should generally limit while eating Mediterranean-style meals. Heavily processed foods. Let's be real: Many, many foods are processed to some degree. A can of beans has been processed, in the sense that the beans have been cooked before being canned. Olive oil has been processed, because olives have been turned into oil. But when we talk about limiting processed foods, this really means avoiding things like frozen meals with tons of sodium. You should also limit soda, desserts and candy. As the adage goes, if the ingredient list includes items that your great-grandparents wouldn't recognize as food, it's probably processed. If you're buying a packaged food that's as close to its whole-food form as possible — such as frozen fruit or veggies with nothing added — you're good to go.

Processed red meat

On the Mediterranean diet, you should minimize your intake of red meat, such as steak. What about processed red meat, such as hot dogs and bacon? You should avoid these foods or limit them as much as possible. A study published in BMJ found that regularly eating red meat, especially processed varieties, was associated with a higher risk of death. Butter. Here's another food that should be limited on the Mediterranean diet. Use olive oil instead, which has many heart health benefits and contains less saturated fat than butter. According to the USDA National Nutrient Database, butter has 7 grams of saturated fat per tablespoon, while olive oil has about 2 grams.

Refined grains

The Mediterranean diet is centered around whole grains, such as farro, millet, couscous and brown rice. With this eating style, you'll generally want to limit your intake of refined grains such as white pasta and white bread.

Alcohol

When you're following the Mediterranean diet, red wine should be your chosen alcoholic drink. This is because red wine offers health benefits, particularly for the heart. But it's important to limit intake of any type of alcohol to up to one drink per day for women, as well as men older than 65, and up to two drinks daily for men age 65 and younger. The amount that counts as a drink is 5 ounces of wine, 12 ounces of beer or 1.5 ounces of 80-proof liquor.

Cucumber Olive Rice

Servings: 8
Cooking Time: 10 Minutes

Ingredients:
- 2 cups rice, rinsed
- 1/2 cup olives, pitted
- 1 cup cucumber, chopped
- 1 tbsp red wine vinegar
- 1 tsp lemon zest, grated
- 1 tbsp fresh lemon juice
- 2 tbsp olive oil
- 2 cups vegetable broth
- 1/2 tsp dried oregano
- 1 red bell pepper, chopped
- 1/2 cup onion, chopped
- 1 tbsp olive oil
- Pepper
- Salt

Directions:
1. Add oil into the inner pot of instant pot and set the pot on sauté mode.
2. Add onion and sauté for 3 minutes.
3. Add bell pepper and oregano and sauté for 1 minute.
4. Add rice and broth and stir well.
5. Seal pot with lid and cook on high for 6 minutes.
6. Once done, allow to release pressure naturally for 10 minutes then release remaining using quick release. Remove lid.

7. Add remaining ingredients and stir everything well to mix. 8. Serve immediately and enjoy it.

Nutrition Info: Calories 229 Fat 5.1 g Carbohydrates 40.2 g Sugar 1.6 g Protein 4.9 g Cholesterol 0 mg

Chorizo-kidney Beans Quinoa Pilaf

Servings: 4
Cooking Time: 35 Minutes

Ingredients:
- ¼ pound dried Spanish chorizo diced (about 2/3 cup)
- ¼ teaspoon red pepper flakes
- ¼ teaspoon smoked paprika
- ½ teaspoon cumin
- ½ teaspoon sea salt
- 1 3/4 cups water
- 1 cup quinoa
- 1 large clove garlic minced
- 1 small red bell pepper finely diced
- 1 small red onion finely diced
- 1 tablespoon tomato paste
- 1 15-ounce can kidney beans rinsed and drained

Directions:
1. Place a nonstick pot on medium high fire and heat for 2 minutes. Add chorizo and sauté for 5 minutes until lightly browned.
2. Stir in peppers and onion. Sauté for 5 minutes.
3. Add tomato paste, red pepper flakes, salt, paprika, cumin, and garlic. Sauté for 2 minutes.
4. Stir in quinoa and mix well. Sauté for 2 minutes.
5. Add water and beans. Mix well. Cover and simmer for 20 minutes or until liquid is fully absorbed.
6. Turn off fire and fluff quinoa. Let it sit for 5 minutes more while uncovered.

7. Serve and enjoy.

Nutrition Info: Calories per serving: 260; Protein: 9.6g; Carbs: 40.9g; Fat: 6.8g

Belly-filling Cajun Rice & Chicken

Servings: 6
Cooking Time: 20 Minutes

Ingredients:
- 1 tablespoon oil
- 1 onion, diced
- 3 cloves of garlic, minced
- 1-pound chicken breasts, sliced
- 1 tablespoon Cajun seasoning
- 1 tablespoon tomato paste
- 2 cups chicken broth
- 1 ½ cups white rice, rinsed
- 1 bell pepper, chopped

Directions:
1. Press the Sauté on the Instant Pot and pour the oil.
2. Sauté the onion and garlic until fragrant.
3. Stir in the chicken breasts and season with Cajun seasoning.
4. Continue cooking for 3 minutes.
5. Add the tomato paste and chicken broth. Dissolve the tomato paste before adding the rice and bell pepper.
6. Close the lid and press the rice button.
7. Once done cooking, do a natural release for 10 minutes.
8. Then, do a quick release.
9. Once cooled, evenly divide into serving size, keep in your preferred container, and refrigerate until ready to eat.

Nutrition Info: Calories per serving: 337; Carbohydrates: 44.3g; Protein: 26.1g; Fat: 5.0g

Chicken And White Bean

Servings: 8
Cooking Time: 70 Minutes

Ingredients:
- 2 tbsp fresh cilantro, chopped
- 2 cups grated Monterey Jack cheese
- 3 cups water
- 1/8 tsp cayenne pepper
- 2 tsp pure chile powder
- 2 tsp ground cumin
- 1 4-oz can chopped green chiles
- 1 cup corn kernels
- 2 15-oz cans shite beans, drained and rinsed
- 2 garlic cloves
- 1 medium onion, diced
- 2 tbsp extra virgin olive oil
- 1 lb. chicken breasts, boneless and skinless

Directions:
1. Slice chicken breasts into ½-inch cubes and with pepper and salt, season it.
2. On high fire, place a large nonstick fry pan and heat oil.
3. Sauté chicken pieces for three to four minutes or until lightly browned.
4. Reduce fire to medium and add garlic and onion.
5. Cook for 5 to 6 minutes or until onions are translucent.
6. Add water, spices, chilies, corn and beans. Bring to a boil.
7. Once boiling, slow fire to a simmer and continue simmering for an hour, uncovered.

8. To serve, garnish with a sprinkling of cilantro and a tablespoon of cheese.

Nutrition Info: Calories per serving: 433; Protein: 30.6g; Carbs: 29.5g; Fat: 21.8g

Quinoa & Black Bean Stuffed Sweet Potatoes

Servings: 8
Cooking Time: 60 Minutes

Ingredients:
- 4 sweet potatoes
- ½ onion, diced
- 1 garlic glove, crushed and diced
- ½ large bell pepper diced (about 2/3 cups)
- Handful of diced cilantro
- ½ cup cooked quinoa
- ½ cup black beans
- 1 tbsp olive oil
- 1 tbsp chili powder
- ½ tbsp cumin
- ½ tsp paprika
- ½ tbsp oregano
- 2 tbsp lime juice
- 2 tbsp honey
- Sprinkle salt
- 1 cup shredded cheddar cheese
- Chopped spring onions, for garnish (optional)

Directions:
1. Preheat oven to 400oF.
2. Wash and scrub outside of potatoes. Poke with fork a few times and then place on parchment paper on cookie sheet. Bake for 40-45 minutes or until it is cooked.

3. While potatoes are baking, sauté onions, garlic, olive oil and spices in a pan on the stove until onions are translucent and soft.

4. In the last 10 minutes while the potatoes are cooking, in a large bowl combine the onion mixture with the beans, quinoa, honey, lime juice, cilantro and ½ cup cheese. Mix well.

5. When potatoes are cooked, remove from oven and let cool slightly. When cool to touch, cut in half (hot dog style) and scoop out most of the insides. Leave a thin ring of potato so that it will hold its shape. You can save the sweet potato guts for another recipe, such as my veggie burgers (recipe posted below).

6. Fill with bean and quinoa mixture. Top with remaining cheddar cheese.

7. (If making this a freezer meal, stop here. Individually wrap potato skins in plastic wrap and place on flat surface to freeze. Once frozen, place all potatoes in large zip lock container or Tupperware.)

8. Return to oven for an additional 10 minutes or until cheese is melted.

Nutrition Info: Calories per serving: 243; Carbs: 37.6g; Protein: 8.5g; Fat: 7.3g

Feta, Eggplant And Sausage Penne

Servings: 6
Cooking Time: 30 Minutes

Ingredients:
- ¼ cup chopped fresh parsley
- ½ cup crumbled feta cheese
- 6 cups hot cooked penne
- 1 14.5oz can diced tomatoes
- ¼ tsp ground black pepper
- 1 tsp dried oregano
- 2 tbsp tomato paste
- 4 garlic cloves, minced
- ½ lb. bulk pork breakfast sausage
- 4 ½ cups cubed peeled eggplant

Directions:
1. On medium high fire, place a nonstick, big fry pan and cook for seven minutes garlic, sausage and eggplant or until eggplants are soft and sausage are lightly browned.
2. Stir in diced tomatoes, black pepper, oregano and tomato paste. Cover and simmer for five minutes while occasionally stirring.
3. Remove pan from fire, stir in pasta and mix well.
4. Transfer to a serving dish, garnish with parsley and cheese before serving.

Nutrition Info: Calories per Serving: 376; Carbs: 50.8g; Protein: 17.8g; Fat: 11.6g

Bell Peppers 'n Tomato-chickpea Rice

Servings: 4
Cooking Time: 35 Minutes

Ingredients:
- 2 tablespoons olive oil
- 1/2 chopped red bell pepper
- 1/2 chopped green bell pepper
- 1/2 chopped yellow pepper
- 1/2 chopped red pepper
- 1 medium onion, chopped
- 1 clove garlic, minced
- 2 cups cooked jasmine rice
- 1 teaspoon tomato paste
- 1 cup chickpeas
- salt to taste
- 1/2 teaspoon paprika
- 1 small tomato, chopped
- Parsley for garnish

Directions:
1. In a large mixing bowl, whisk well olive oil, garlic, tomato paste, and paprika. Season with salt generously.
2. Mix in rice and toss well to coat in the dressing.
3. Add remaining ingredients and toss well to mix.
4. Let salad rest to allow flavors to mix for 15 minutes.
5. Toss one more time and adjust salt to taste if needed.
6. Garnish with parsley and serve.

Nutrition Info: Calories per serving: 490; Carbs: 93.0g; Protein: 10.0g; Fat: 8.0g

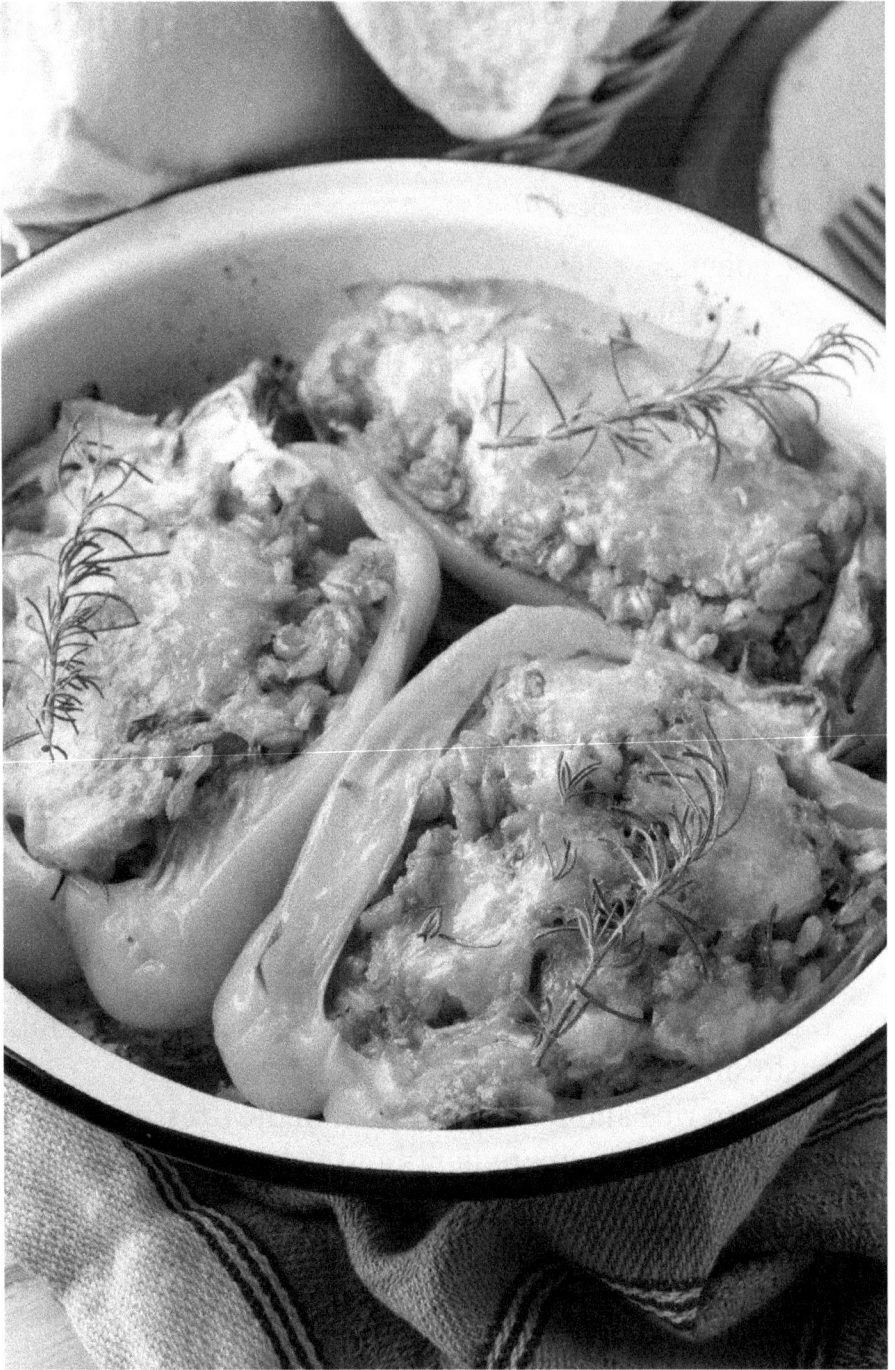

Lip Smacking Chicken Tetrazzini

Servings: 8
Cooking Time: 3 Hours

Ingredients:
- Toasted French bread slices
- ¾ cup thinly sliced green onion
- 2/3 cup grated parmesan cheese
- 10 oz dried spaghetti or linguine, cooked and drained
- ¼ tsp ground nutmeg
- ¼ tsp ground black pepper
- 2 tbsp dry sherry
- ¼ cup chicken broth or water
- 1 16 oz jar of Alfredo pasta sauce
- 2 4.5oz jars of sliced mushrooms, drained
- 2.5 lbs. skinless chicken breasts cut into ½ inch slices

Directions:
1. In a slow cooker, mix mushrooms and chicken.
2. In a bowl, mix well nutmeg, pepper, sherry, broth and alfredo sauce before pouring over chicken and mushrooms.
3. Set on high heat, cover and cook for two to three hours.
4. Once chicken is cooked, pour over pasta, garnish with green onion and serve with French bread on the side.

Nutrition Info: Calories per Serving: 505; Carbs: 24.7g; Protein: 35.1g; Fat: 30.2g

Spaghetti In Lemon Avocado White Sauce

Servings: 6
Cooking Time: 30 Minutes

Ingredients:
- Freshly ground black pepper
- Zest and juice of 1 lemon
- 1 avocado, pitted and peeled
- 1-pound spaghetti
- Salt
- 1 tbsp Olive oil
- 8 oz small shrimp, shelled and deveined
- ¼ cup dry white wine
- 1 large onion, finely sliced

Directions:
1. Let a big pot of water boil. Once boiling add the spaghetti or pasta and cook following manufacturer's instructions until al dente. Drain and set aside.
2. In a large fry pan, over medium fire sauté wine and onions for ten minutes or until onions are translucent and soft.
3. Add the shrimps into the fry pan and increase fire to high while constantly sautéing until shrimps are cooked around five minutes. Turn the fire off. Season with salt and add the oil right away. Then quickly toss in the cooked pasta, mix well.

4. In a blender, until smooth, puree the lemon juice and avocado. Pour into the fry pan of pasta, combine well. Garnish with pepper and lemon zest then serve.

Nutrition Info: Calories per Serving: 206; Carbs: 26.3g; Protein: 10.2g; Fat: 8.0g

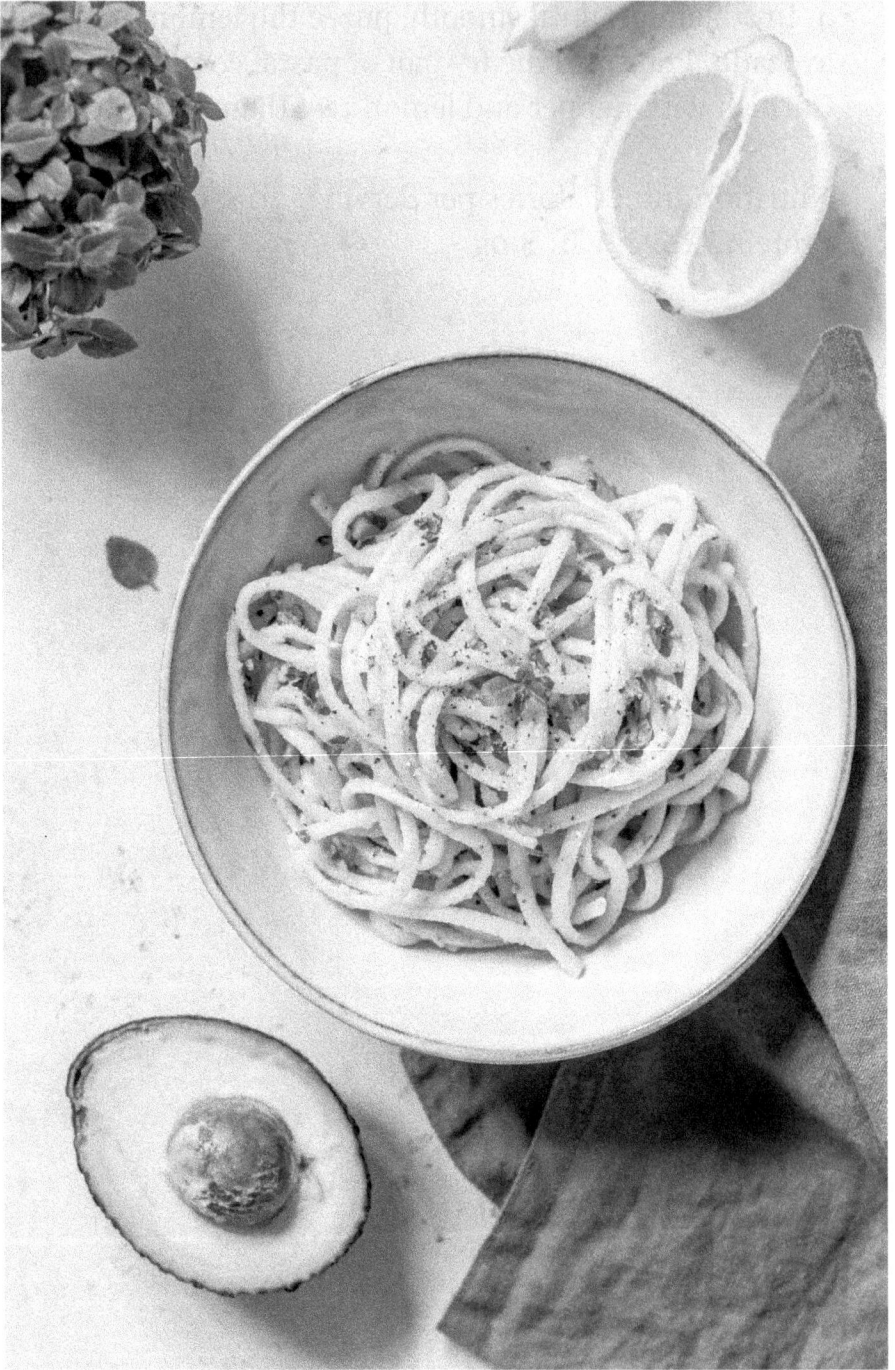

Kidney Beans And Beet Salad

Servings: 4
Cooking Time: 15 Minutes

Ingredients:
- 1 14.5-ounce can kidney beans, drained and rinsed
- 1 tablespoon pomegranate syrup or juice
- 2 tablespoons olive oil
- 4 beets, scrubbed and stems removed
- 4 green onions, chopped
- Juice of 1 lemon
- Salt and pepper to taste

Directions:
1. Bring a pot of water to boil and add beets. Simmer for 10 minutes or until tender. Drain beets and place in ice bath for 5 minutes.
2. Peel bets and slice in halves.
3. Toss to mix the pomegranate syrup, olive oil, lemon juice, green onions, and kidney beans in a salad bowl.
4. Stir in beets. Season with pepper and salt to taste.
5. Serve and enjoy.

Nutrition Info: Calories per serving: 175; Protein: 6.0g; Carbs: 22.0g; Fat: 7.0g

Filling Macaroni Soup

Servings: 6
Cooking Time: 45 Minutes

Ingredients:
- 1 cup of minced beef or chicken or a combination of both
- 1 cup carrots, diced
- 1 cup milk
- ½ medium onion, sliced thinly
- 3 garlic cloves, minced
- Salt and pepper to taste
- 2 cups broth (chicken, vegetable or beef)
- ½ tbsp olive oil
- 1 cup uncooked whole wheat pasta like macaroni, shells, even angel hair broken to pieces
- 1 cup water

Directions:
1. In a heavy bottomed pot on medium high fire heat oil.
2. Add garlic and sauté for a minute or two until fragrant but not browned.
3. Add onions and sauté for 3 minutes or until soft and translucent.
4. Add a cup of minced meat. You can also use whatever leftover frozen meat you have.
5. Sauté the meat well until cooked around 8 minutes. While sautéing, season meat with pepper and salt.
6. Add water and broth and bring to a boil.
7. Once boiling, add pasta. I use any leftover pasta that I have in the pantry. If all you have left is spaghetti, lasagna,

angel hair or fettuccine, just break them into pieces—around 1-inch in length before adding to the pot.

8. Slow fire to a simmer and cook while covered until pasta is soft.

9. Halfway through cooking the pasta, around 8 minutes I add the carrots.

10. Once the pasta is soft, turn off fire and add milk.

11. Mix well and season to taste again if needed.

12. Serve and enjoy.

Nutrition Info: Calories per Serving: 125; Carbs: 11.4g; Protein: 10.1g; Fat: 4.3g

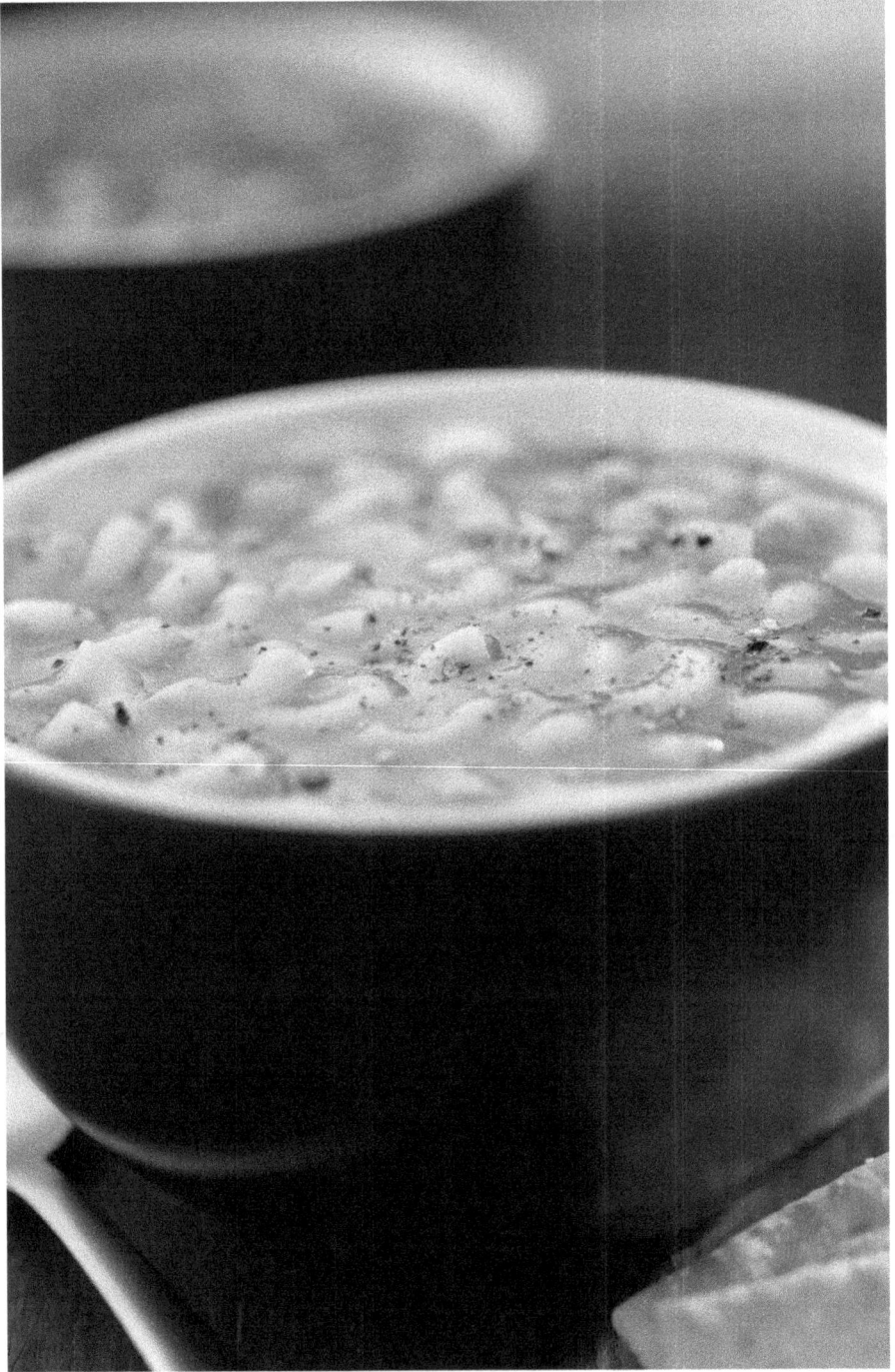

Simple Penne Antipasto

Servings: 4
Cooking Time: 15 Minutes

Ingredients:
- ¼ cup pine nuts, toasted
- ½ cup grated Parmigiano-Reggiano cheese, divided
- 8oz penne pasta, cooked and drained
- 1 6oz jar drained, sliced, marinated and quartered artichoke hearts 1 7 oz jar drained and chopped sun-dried tomato halves packed in oil 3 oz chopped prosciutto
- 1/3 cup pesto
- ½ cup pitted and chopped Kalamata olives
- 1 medium red bell pepper

Directions:
1. Slice bell pepper, discard membranes, seeds and stem. On a foiled lined baking sheet, place bell pepper halves, press down by hand and broil in oven for eight minutes. Remove from oven, put in a sealed bag for 5 minutes before peeling and chopping.
2. Place chopped bell pepper in a bowl and mix in artichokes, tomatoes, prosciutto, pesto and olives.
3. Toss in ¼ cup cheese and pasta. Transfer to a serving dish and garnish with ¼ cup cheese and pine nuts. Serve and enjoy!

Nutrition Info: Calories per Serving: 606; Carbs: 70.3g; Protein: 27.2g; Fat: 27.6g

Squash And Eggplant Casserole

Servings: 2
Cooking Time: 45 Minutes

Ingredients:
- ½ cup dry white wine
- 1 eggplant, halved and cut to 1-inch slices
- 1 large onion, cut into wedges
- 1 red bell pepper, seeded and cut to julienned strips
- 1 small butternut squash, cut into 1-inch slices
- 1 tbsp olive oil
- 12 baby corn
- 2 cups low sodium vegetable broth
- Salt and pepper to taste
- ¼ cup parmesan cheese, grated
- 1 cup instant polenta
- 2 tbsp fresh oregano, chopped
- 1 garlic clove, chopped
- 2 tbsp slivered almonds
- 5 tbsp parsley, chopped
- Grated zest of 1 lemon

Directions:
1. Preheat the oven to 350 degrees Fahrenheit.
2. In a casserole, heat the oil and add the onion wedges and baby corn. Sauté over medium high heat for five minutes. Stir occasionally to prevent the onions and baby corn from sticking at the bottom of the pan.
3. Add the butternut squash to the casserole and toss the vegetables. Add the eggplants and the red pepper.
4. Cover the vegetables and cook over low to medium heat.

5. Cook for about ten minutes before adding the wine. Let the wine sizzle
before stirring in the broth. Bring to a boil and cook in the oven for 30 minutes.

6. While the casserole is cooking inside the oven, make the topping by spreading the slivered almonds on a baking tray and toasting under the grill until they are lightly browned.

7. Place the toasted almonds in a small bowl and mix the remaining ingredients for the toppings.

8. Prepare the polenta. In a large saucepan, bring 3 cups of water to boil over high heat.

9. Add the polenta and continue whisking until it absorbs all the water.

10. Reduce the heat to medium until the polenta is thick. Add the parmesan cheese and oregano.

11. Serve the polenta on plates and add the casserole on top. Sprinkle the toppings on top.

Nutrition Info: Calories per Serving: 579.3; Carbs: 79.2g; Protein: 22.2g; Fat: 19.3g

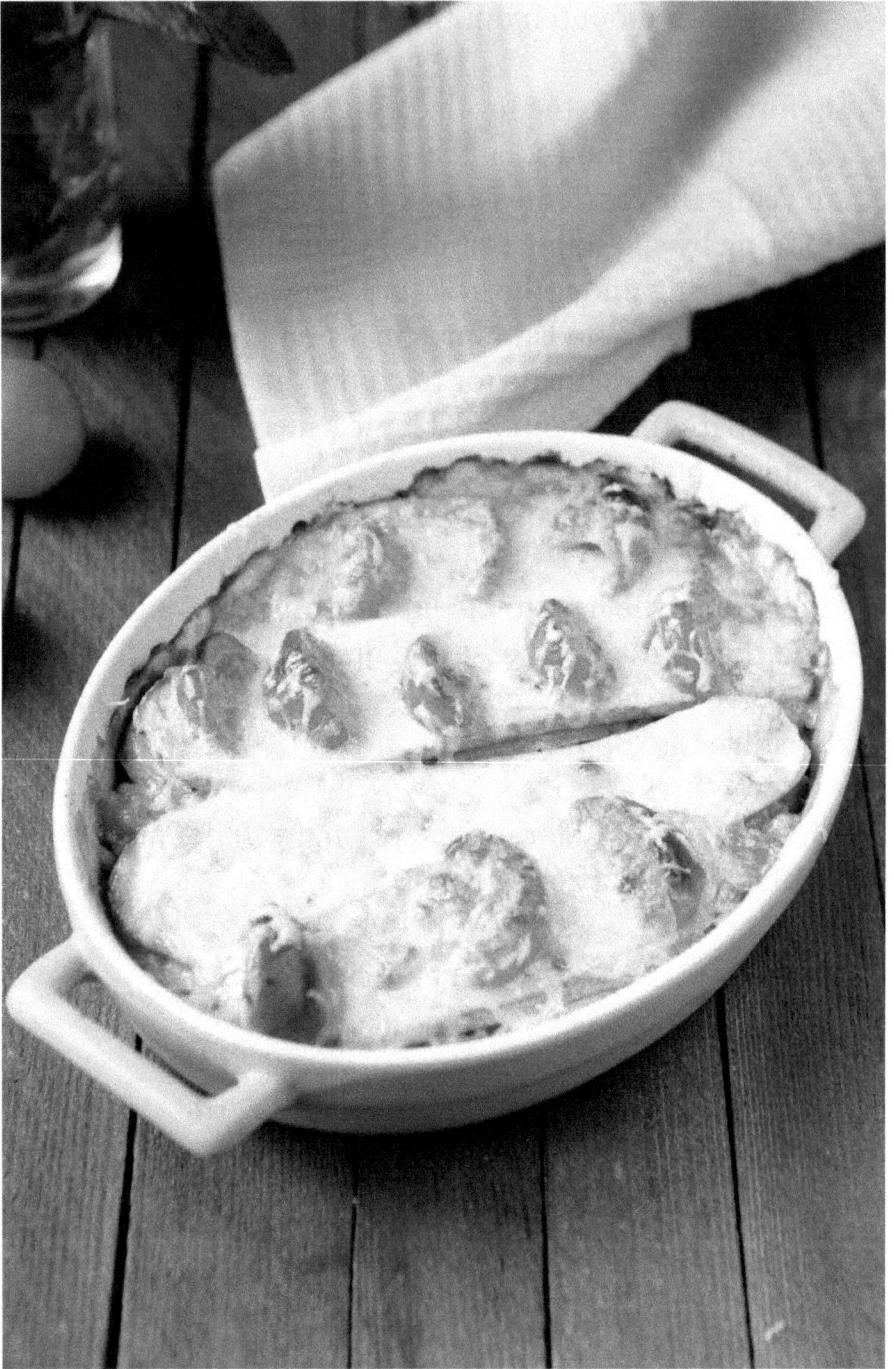

Blue Cheese And Grains Salad

Servings: 4
Cooking Time: 40 Minutes

Ingredients:
- ¼ cup thinly sliced scallions
- ½ cup millet, rinsed
- ½ cup quinoa, rinsed
- 1 ½ tsp olive oil
- 1 Bartlett pear, cored and diced
- 1/8 tsp ground black pepper
- 2 cloves garlic, minced
- 2 oz blue cheese
- 2 tbsp fresh lemon juice
- 2 tsp dried rosemary
- 4 4-oz boneless, skinless chicken breasts
- 6 oz baby spinach
- olive oil cooking spray
- ¼ cup fresh raspberries
- 1 tbsp pure maple syrup
- 1 tsp fresh thyme leaf
- 2 tbsp grainy mustard
- 6 tbsp balsamic vinegar

Directions:
1. Bring millet, quinoa, and 2 ¼ cups water on a small saucepan to a boil. Once boiling, slow fire to a simmer and stir once. Cover and cook until water is fully absorbed and grains are soft around 15 minutes. Turn off fire, fluff grains with a fork and set aside to cool a bit.

2. Arrange one oven rack to highest position and preheat broiler. Line a baking sheet with foil, and grease with cooking spray.

3. Whisk well pepper, oil, rosemary, lemon juice and garlic. Rub onto chicken.

4. Place chicken on prepared pan, pop into the broiler and broil until juices run clear and no longer pin inside around 12 minutes.

5. Meanwhile, make the dressing by combining all ingredients in a blender. Blend until smooth.

6. Remove chicken from oven, cool slightly before cutting into strips, against the grain.

7. To assemble, place grains in a large salad bowl. Add in dressing and spinach, toss to mix well.

8. Add scallions and pear, mix gently and evenly divide into four plates. Top each salad with cheese and chicken.

9. Serve and enjoy.

Nutrition Info: Calories per Serving: 530.4; Carbs: 77g; Protein: 21.4g; Fat: 15.2g

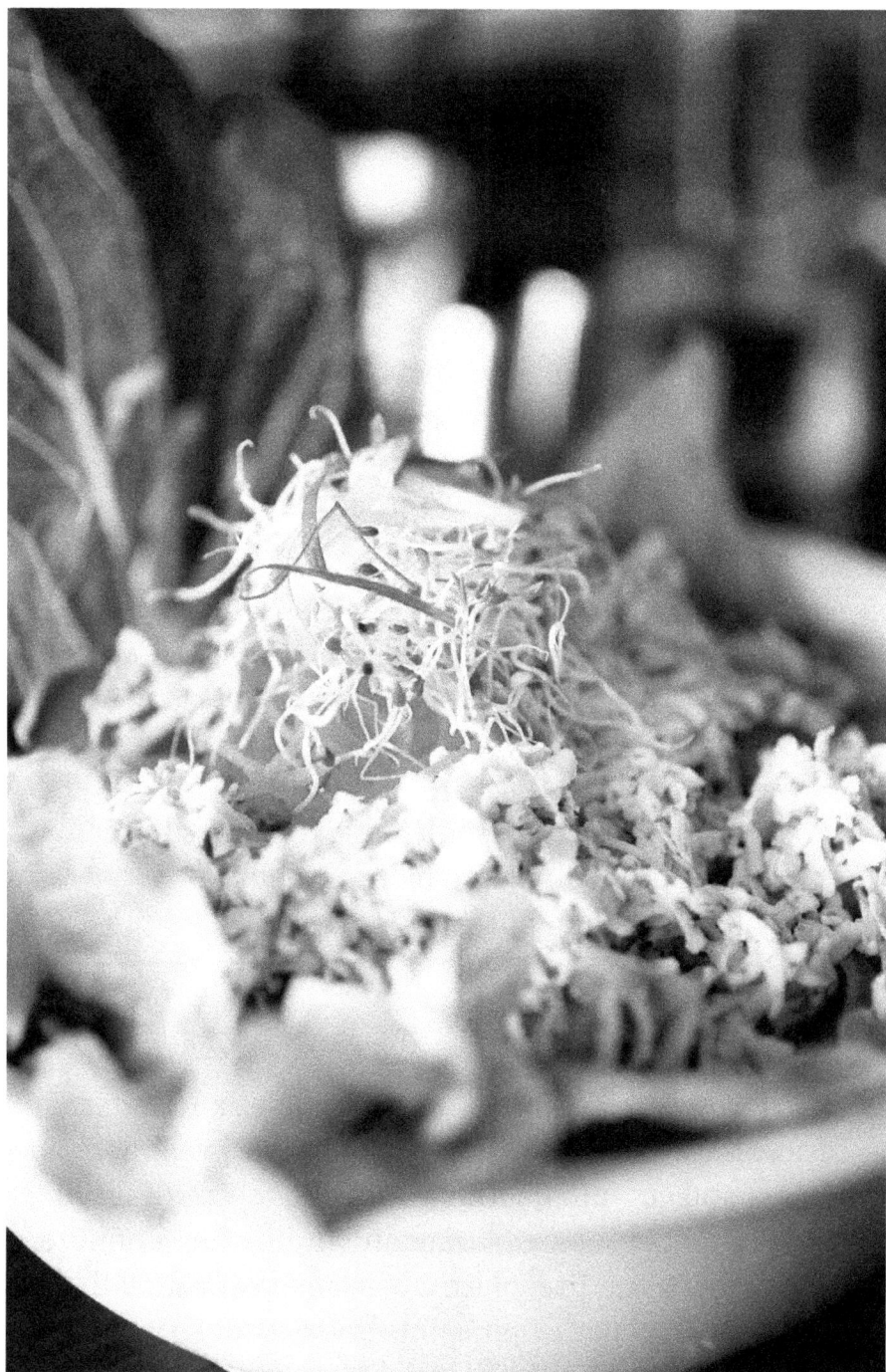

Creamy Artichoke Lasagna

Servings: 8
Cooking Time: 70 Minutes

Ingredients:
- 1 cup shredded mozzarella cheese
- 2 cups light cream
- ¼ cup all-purpose flour
- 1 cup vegetable broth
- ¾ tsp salt
- 1 egg
- 1 cup snipped fresh basil
- 1 cup finely shredded Parmesan cheese
- 1 15-oz carton ricotta cheese
- 4 cloves garlic, minced
- ½ cup pine nuts
- 3 tbsp olive oil
- 9 dried lasagna noodles, cooked, rinsed in cold water and drained 15 fresh baby artichokes
- ¼ cup lemon juice
- 3 cups water

Directions:
1. Prepare in a medium bowl lemon juice and water. Put aside. Slice off artichoke base and remove yellowed outer leaves and cut into quarters. Immediately soak sliced artichokes in prepared liquid and drain after a minute.
2. Over medium fire, place a big saucepan with 2 tbsp oil and fry half of garlic, pine nuts and artichokes. Stir frequently and cook until artichokes are soft around ten minutes. Turn off fire and transfer mixture to a big bowl

and quickly stir in salt, egg, ½ cup of basil, ½ cup of parmesan cheese and ricotta cheese. Mix thoroughly.

3. In a small bowl mix flour and broth. In same pan, add 1 tbsp oil and fry remaining garlic for half a minute. Add light cream and flour mixture. Stir constantly and cook until thickened. Remove from fire and stir in ½ cup of basil.

4. In a separate bowl mix ½ cup parmesan and mozzarella cheese.

5. Assemble the lasagna by layering the following in a greased rectangular glass dish: lasagna, 1/3 of artichoke mixture, 1/3 of sauce, sprinkle with the dried cheeses and repeat layering procedure until all ingredients are used up.

6. For forty minutes, bake lasagna in a preheated oven of 350oF. Remove lasagna from oven and before serving, let it stand for fifteen minutes.

Nutrition Info: Calories per Serving: 425; Carbs: 41.4g; Protein: 21.3g; Fat: 19.8g

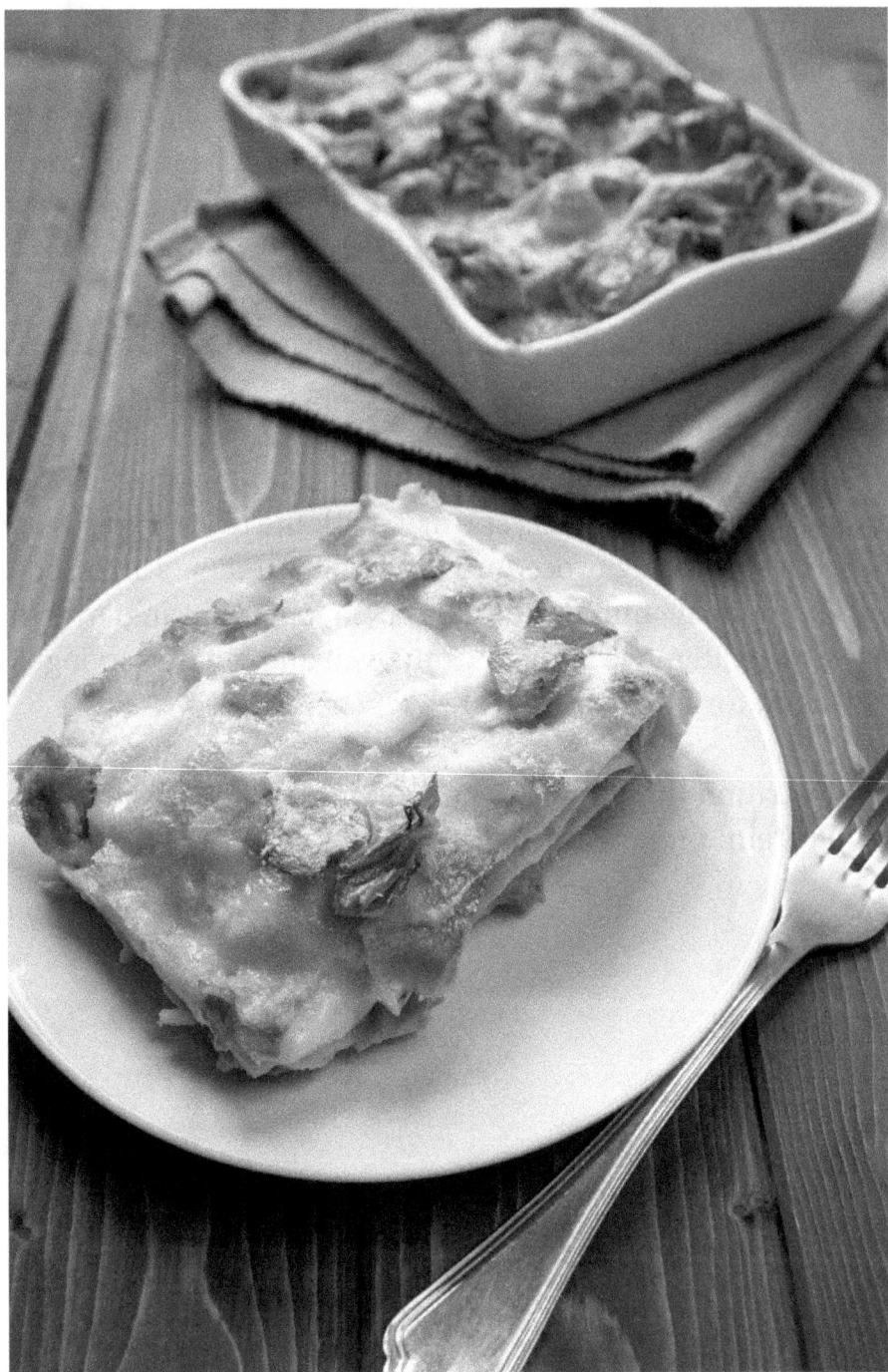

Brown Rice Pilaf With Butternut Squash

Servings: 8
Cooking Time: 50 Minutes

Ingredients:
- Pepper to taste
- A pinch of cinnamon
- 1 tsp salt
- 2 tbsp chopped fresh oregano
- ½ cup chopped fennel fronds
- ½ cup white wine
- 1 ¾ cups water + 2 tbsp, divided
- 1 cup instant or parboiled brown rice
- 1 tbsp tomato paste
- 1 garlic clove, minced
- 1 large onion, finely chopped
- 3 tbsp extra virgin olive oil
- 2 lbs. butternut squash, peeled, halved and seeded

Directions:
1. In a large hole grater, grate squash.
2. On medium low fire, place a large nonstick skillet and heat oil for 2 minutes.
3. Add garlic and onions. Sauté for 8 minutes or until lightly colored and soft.
4. Add 2 tbsp water and tomato paste. Stir well to combine and cook for 3 minutes.
5. Add rice, mix well to coat in mixture and cook for 5 minutes while stirring frequently.

6. If needed, add squash in batches until it has wilted so that you can cover pan.

7. Add remaining water and increase fire to medium high.

8. Add wine, cover and boil. Once boiling, lower fire to a simmer and cook for 20 to 25 minutes or until liquid is fully absorbed.

9. Stir in pepper, cinnamon, salt, oregano, and fennel fronds. 10. Turn off fire, cover and let it stand for 5 minutes before serving.

Nutrition Info: Calories per Serving: 147; Carbs: 22.1g; Protein: 2.3g; Fat: 5.5g

Cranberry And Roasted Squash Delight

Servings: 8
Cooking Time: 60 Minutes
Ingredients:

- ¼ cup chopped walnuts
- ¼ tsp thyme
- ½ tbsp chopped Italian parsley
- 1 cup diced onion
- 1 cup fresh cranberries
- 1 small orange, peeled and segmented
- 2 tsp canola oil, divided
- 4 cups cooked wild rice
- 4 cups diced winter squash, peeled and cut into ½-inch cubes Pepper to taste

Directions:

1. Grease roasting pan with cooking spray and preheat oven to 400oF.
2. In prepped roasting pan place squash cubes, add a teaspoon of oil and toss to coat. Place in oven and roast until lightly browned, around 40 minutes.
3. On medium high fire, place a nonstick fry pan and heat remaining oil. Once hot, add onions and sauté until lightly browned and tender, around 5 minutes.
4. Add cranberries and continue stir frying for a minute.
5. Add remaining ingredients into pan and cook until heated through around four to five minutes.
6. Best served warm.

Nutrition Info: Calories per Serving: 166.2; Protein: 4.8g; Carbs: 29.1g; Fat: 3.4g

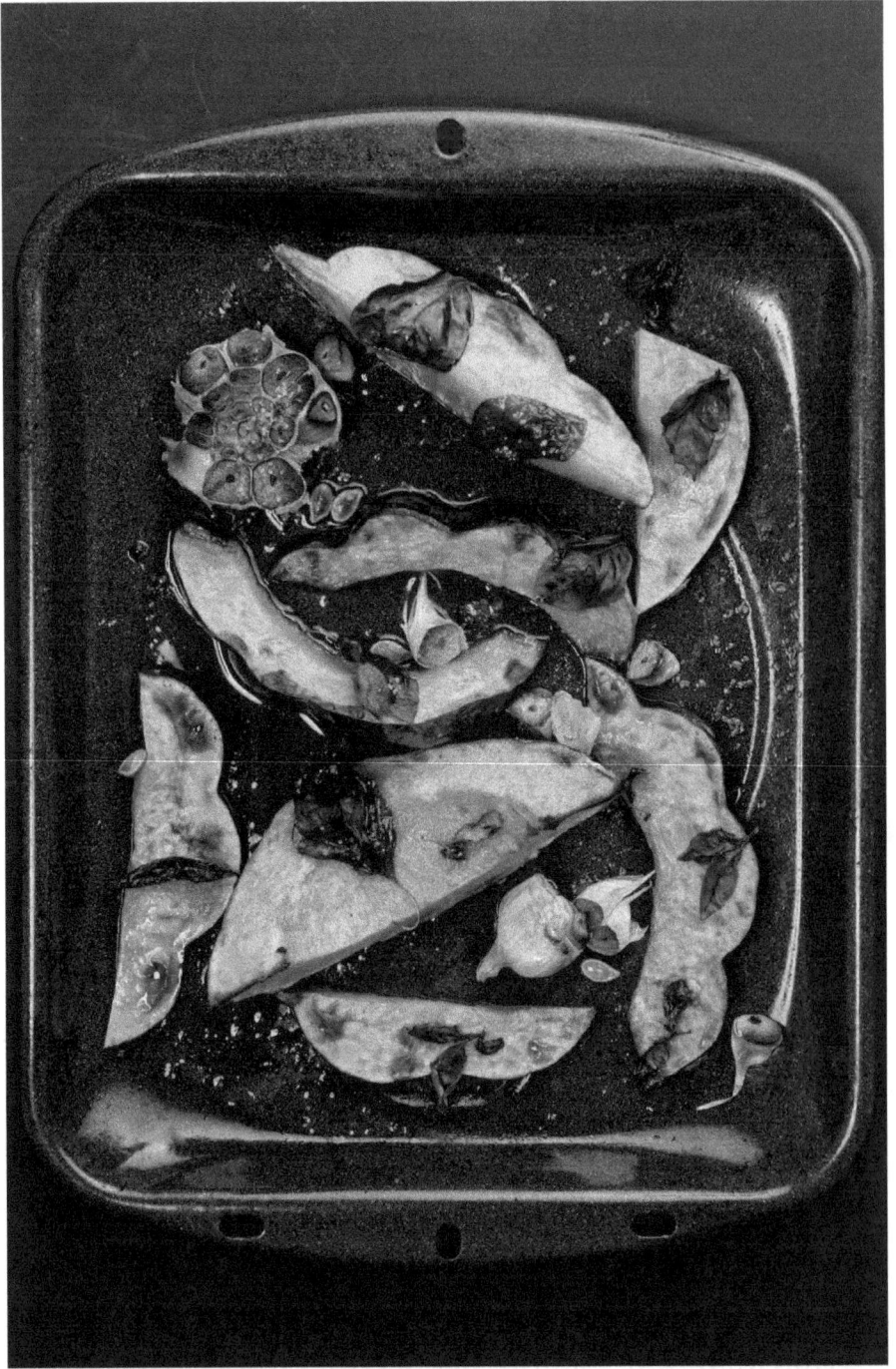

Spanish Rice Casserole With Cheesy Beef

Servings: 2
Cooking Time: 32 Minutes

Ingredients:
- 2 tablespoons chopped green bell pepper
- 1/4 teaspoon Worcestershire sauce
- 1/4 teaspoon ground cumin
- 1/4 cup shredded Cheddar cheese
- 1/4 cup finely chopped onion
- 1/4 cup chile sauce
- 1/3 cup uncooked long grain rice
- 1/2-pound lean ground beef
- 1/2 teaspoon salt
- 1/2 teaspoon brown sugar
- 1/2 pinch ground black pepper
- 1/2 cup water
- 1/2 (14.5 ounce) can canned tomatoes
- 1 tablespoon chopped fresh cilantro

Directions:
1. Place a nonstick saucepan on medium fire and brown beef for 10 minutes while crumbling beef. Discard fat.
2. Stir in pepper, Worcestershire sauce, cumin, brown sugar, salt, chile sauce, rice, water, tomatoes, green bell pepper, and onion. Mix well and cook for 10 minutes until blended and a bit tender.
3. Transfer to an ovenproof casserole and press down firmly. Sprinkle cheese on top and cook for 7 minutes at

400F preheated oven. Broil for 3 minutes until top is lightly browned.

4. Serve and enjoy with chopped cilantro.

Nutrition Info: Calories per serving: 460; Carbohydrates: 35.8g; Protein: 37.8g; Fat: 17.9g

Kidney Bean And Parsley-lemon Salad

Servings: 6
Cooking Time: 0 Minutes

Ingredients:
- ¼ cup lemon juice (about 1 ½ lemons)
- ¼ cup olive oil
- ¾ cup chopped fresh parsley
- ¾ teaspoon salt
- 1 can (15 ounces) chickpeas, rinsed and drained, or 1 ½ cups cooked chickpeas
- 1 medium cucumber, peeled, seeded and diced
- 1 small red onion, diced
- 2 cans (15 ounces each) red kidney beans, rinsed and drained, or 3 cups cooked kidney beans
- 2 stalks celery, sliced in half or thirds lengthwise and chopped 2 tablespoons chopped fresh dill or mint
- 3 cloves garlic, pressed or minced
- Small pinch red pepper flakes

Directions:
1. Whisk well in a small bowl the pepper flakes, salt, garlic, and lemon juice until emulsified.
2. In a serving bowl, combine the prepared kidney beans, chickpeas, onion, celery, cucumber, parsley and dill (or mint).
3. Drizzle salad with the dressing and toss well to coat.
4. Serve and enjoy.

Nutrition Info: Calories per serving: 228; Protein: 8.5g; Carbs: 26.2g; Fat: 11.0g

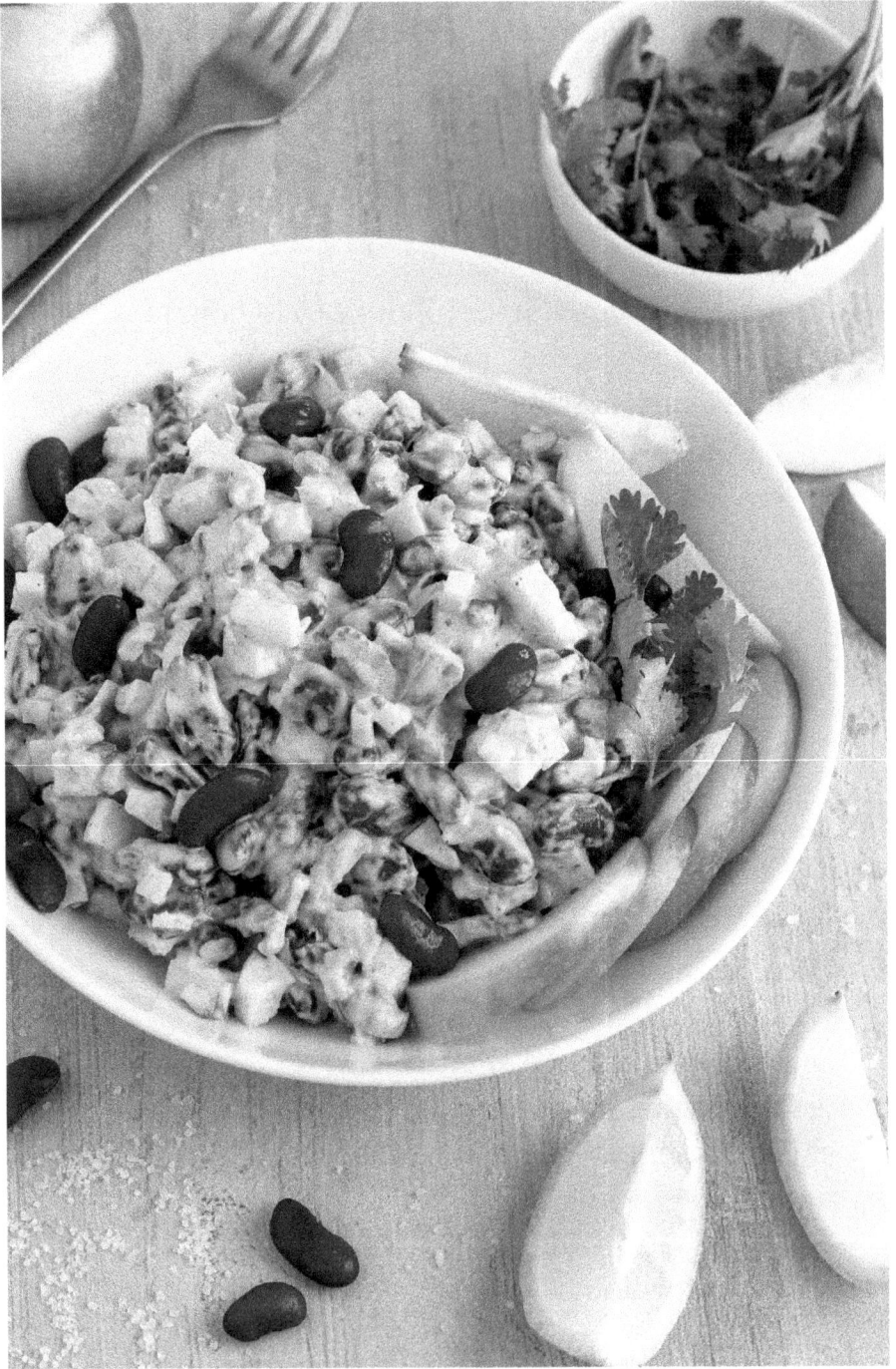

Italian White Bean Soup

Servings: 4
Cooking Time: 50 Minutes

Ingredients:
- 1 (14 ounce) can chicken broth
- 1 bunch fresh spinach, rinsed and thinly sliced
- 1 clove garlic, minced
- 1 stalk celery, chopped
- 1 tablespoon lemon juice
- 1 tablespoon vegetable oil
- 1 onion, chopped
- 1/4 teaspoon ground black pepper
- 1/8 teaspoon dried thyme
- 2 (16 ounce) cans white kidney beans, rinsed and drained
- 2 cups water

Directions:
1. Place a pot on medium high fire and heat pot for a minute. Add oil and heat for another minute.
2. Stir in celery and onion. Sauté for 7 minutes.
3. Stir in garlic and cook for another minute.
4. Add water, thyme, pepper, chicken broth, and beans. Cover and simmer for 15 minutes.
5. Remove 2 cups of the bean and celery mixture with a slotted spoon and set aside.
6. With an immersion blender, puree remaining soup in pot until smooth and creamy.

7. Return the 2 cups of bean mixture. Stir in spinach and lemon juice. Cook for 2 minutes until heated through and spinach is wilted.

8. Serve and enjoy.

Nutrition Info: Calories per serving: 245; Protein: 12.0g; Carbs: 38.1g; Fat: 4.9g

Mexican Quinoa Bake

Servings: 4
Cooking Time: 40 Minutes

Ingredients:

- 3 cups sweet potato, peeled, diced very small (about 1 large sweet potato)
- 2 cups cooked quinoa
- 1 cup shredded sharp cheddar cheese
- 2 Tbs chili powder
- T Tbs paprika
- 1 1/4 cup salsa of your choice
- 1 red bell pepper, diced
- 1 large carrot, diced
- 3 Tbs canned green chiles
- 1 small onion, diced
- 3 garlic cloves, minced
- 2 cups cooked black beans

Directions:
1. Preheat oven to 400F.
2. Dice, chop, measure and prep all ingredients.
3. Combine all ingredients in one big bowl and toss ingredients well.
4. Spray a 9 X 13-inch pan with cooking spray and pour all ingredients in.
5. Bake for 35-40 minutes or until sweet potato pieces are slightly mushy, cheese is melted and items are heated all the way through.
6. Let sit for about 5 minutes, scoop into bowls and enjoy!

Nutrition Info: Calories per serving: 414; Carbs: 56.6g; Protein: 22.0g; Fat: 13.0g

Citrus Quinoa & Chickpea Salad

Servings: 4
Cooking Time: 0 Minutes

Ingredients:
- 2 cups cooked quinoa
- 1 can chickpeas, drained & rinsed
- 1 ripe avocado, diced
- 1 red bell pepper, diced
- 1/2 red onion, diced
- 1/4 cup lime juice
- 1/2 tbsp garlic powder
- 1/2 tbsp paprika
- 1/4-1/2 cup chopped cilantro
- 1 tbsp chopped jalapenos
- Sea salt to taste

Directions:
1. Add all ingredients in a large bowl and mix well.
2. Enjoy right away or refrigerate for later.

Nutrition Info: Calories per serving: 300; Carbs: 43.5g;
Protein: 10.3g; Fat: 10.9g

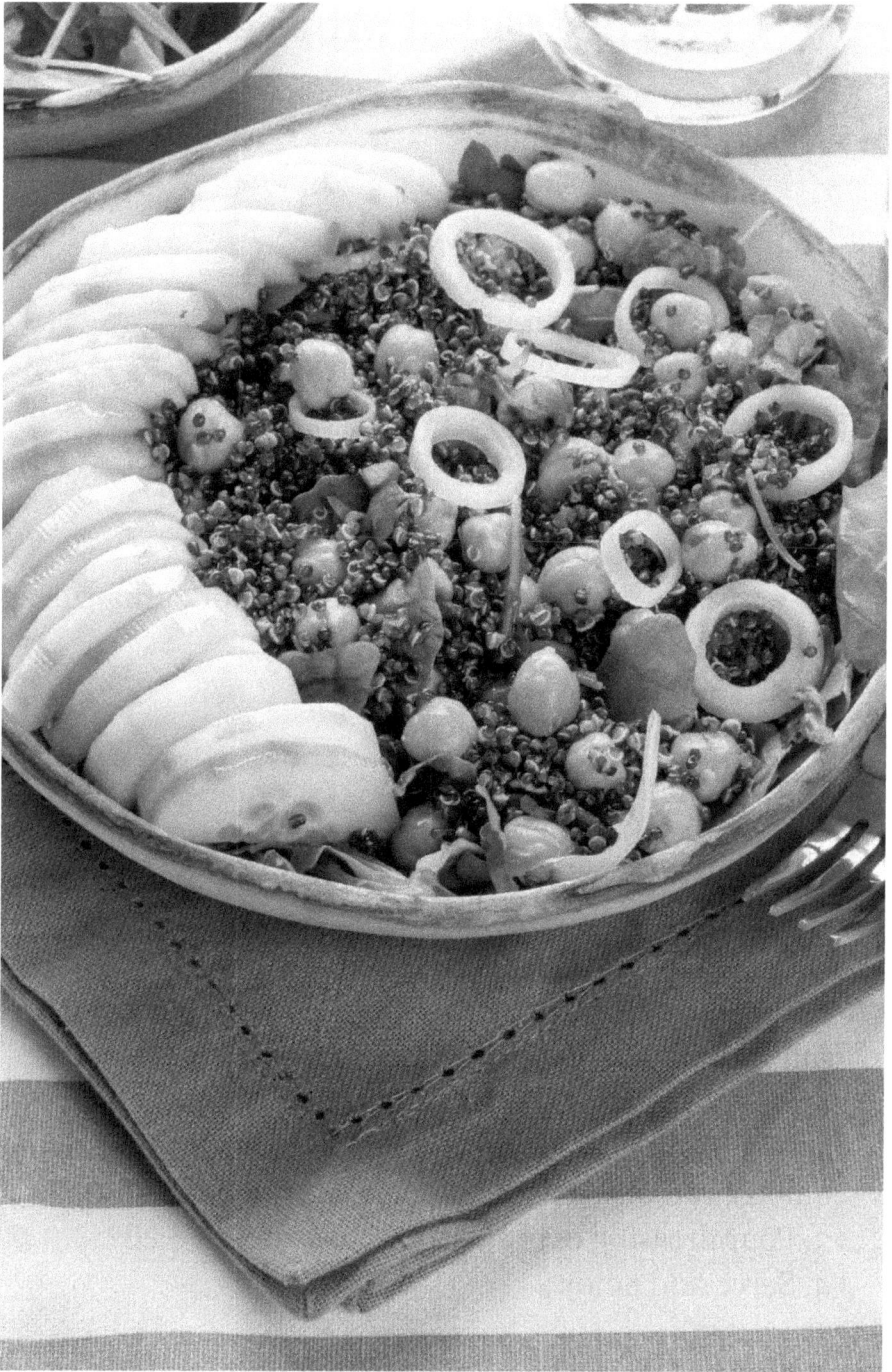

Chickpea Salad Moroccan Style

Servings: 6
Cooking Time: 0 Minutes

Ingredients:
- 1/3 cup crumbled low-fat feta cheese
- ¼ cup fresh mint, chopped
- ¼ cup fresh cilantro, chopped
- 1 red bell pepper, diced
- 2 plum tomatoes, diced
- 3 green onions, sliced thinly
- 1 large carrot, peeled and julienned
- 3 cups BPA free canned chickpeas or garbanzo beans
- Pinch of cayenne pepper
- ¼ tsp salt
- ¼ tsp pepper
- 2 tsp ground cumin
- 3 tbsp fresh lemon juice
- 3 tbsp olive oil

Directions:
1. Make the dressing by whisking cayenne, black pepper, salt, cumin, lemon juice and oil in a small bowl and set aside.
2. Mix together feta, mint, cilantro, red pepper, tomatoes, onions, carrots and chickpeas in a large salad bowl.
3. Pour dressing over salad and toss to coat well.
4. Serve and enjoy.

Nutrition Info: Calories per serving: 300; Protein: 13.2g; Carbs: 35.4g; Fat: 12.8g

Garlicky Peas And Clams On Veggie Spiral

Servings: 4
Cooking Time: 15 Minutes

Ingredients:
- 2 tbsp chopped fresh basil
- ½ cup pre-shredded Parmesan cheese
- 1 cup frozen green peas
- ¼ tsp crushed red pepper
- ¼ cup dry white wine
- 1 cup organic vegetable broth
- 3 cans chopped clams, clams and juice separated
- 1 ½ tsp bottled minced garlic
- 2 tbsp olive oil
- 6 cups zucchini, spiral

Directions:
1. Bring a pot of water to a rolling boil and blanch zucchini for 4 minutes on high fire. Drain and let stand for a couple of minutes to continue cooking.
2. On medium high fire, add a large nonstick saucepan and heat oil. Add and sauté for a minute the garlic. Pour in wine, broth and clam juice.
3. Once liquid is boiling, low fire to a simmer and add pepper. Continue cooking and stirring for 5 minutes.
4. Add peas and clams, cook until heated through or around two minutes.
5. Toss in zucchini, mix well. Cook until heated through.

6. Add basil and cheese, toss to mix well then remove from fire.

7. Transfer equally to four serving bowls and enjoy.

Nutrition Info: Calories per Serving: 210; Carbs: 24.0g; Protein: 8.5g; Fat: 9.2g

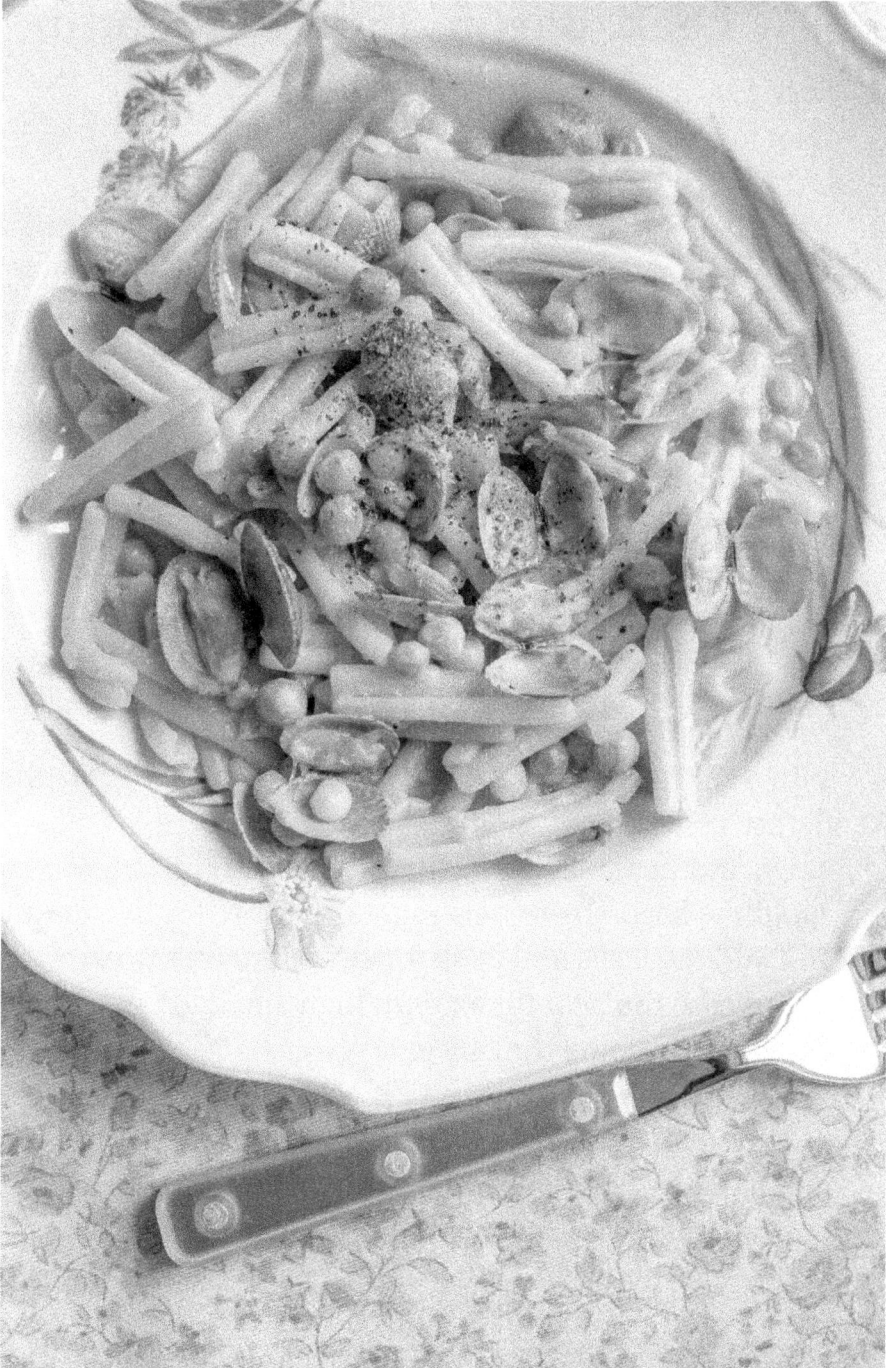

Leek, Bacon And Pea Risotto

Servings: 4
Cooking Time: 60 Minutes

Ingredients:
- Salt and pepper to taste
- 2 tbsp fresh lemon juice
- ½ cup grated parmesan cheese
- ¾ cup frozen peas
- 1 cup dry white wine
- 2 ½ cups Arborio rice
- 4 slices bacon (cut into strips)
- 12 cups low sodium chicken broth
- 2 leeks cut lengthwise

Directions:
1. In a saucepan, bring the broth to a simmer over medium flame.
2. On another skillet, cook bacon and stir continuously to avoid the bacon from burning. Cook more for five minutes and add the leeks and cook for two more minutes.
3. Increase the heat to medium high and add the rice until the grains become translucent.
4. Add the wine and stir until it evaporates.
5. Add 1 cup of broth to the mixture and reduce the heat to medium low. Stir constantly for two minutes.
6. Gradually add the remaining broth until the rice becomes al dente and it becomes creamy.
7. Add the peas and the rest of the broth.
8. Remove the skillet or turn off the heat and add the Parmesan cheese.

9. Cover the skillet and let the cheese melt. Season the risotto with lemon juice, salt and pepper.
10. Serve the risotto with more parmesan cheese.

Nutrition Info: Calories per Serving: 742; Carbs: 57.6g; Protein: 38.67g; Fat: 39.6g

Chickpea Fried Eggplant Salad

Servings: 4
Cooking Time: 10 Minutes

Ingredients:
- 1 cup chopped dill
- 1 cup chopped parsley
- 1 cup cooked or canned chickpeas, drained
- 1 large eggplant, thinly sliced (no more than 1/4 inch in thickness) 1 small red onion, sliced in 1/2 moons
- 1/2 English cucumber, diced
- 3 Roma tomatoes, diced
- 3 tbsp Za'atar spice, divided
- oil for frying, preferably extra virgin olive oil
- Salt
- 1 large lime, juice of
- 1/3 cup extra virgin olive oil
- 1–2 garlic cloves, minced
- Salt & Pepper to taste

Directions:
1. On a baking sheet, spread out sliced eggplant and season with salt generously. Let it sit for 30 minutes. Then pat dry with paper towel.
2. Place a small pot on medium high fire and fill halfway with oil. Heat oil for 5 minutes. Fry eggplant in batches until golden brown, around 3 minutes per side. Place cooked eggplants on a paper towel lined plate.
3. Once eggplants have cooled, assemble the eggplant on a serving dish. Sprinkle with 1 tbsp of Za'atar.

4. Mix dill, parsley, red onions, chickpeas, cucumbers, and tomatoes in a large salad bowl. Sprinkle remaining Za'atar and gently toss to mix.

5. Whisk well the vinaigrette ingredients in a small bowl. Drizzle 2 tbsp of the dressing over the fried eggplant. Add remaining dressing over the chickpea salad and mix.

6. Add the chickpea salad to the serving dish with the fried eggplant.

7. Serve and enjoy.

Nutrition Info: Calories per serving: 642; Protein: 16.6g; Carbs: 25.9g; Fat: 44.0g

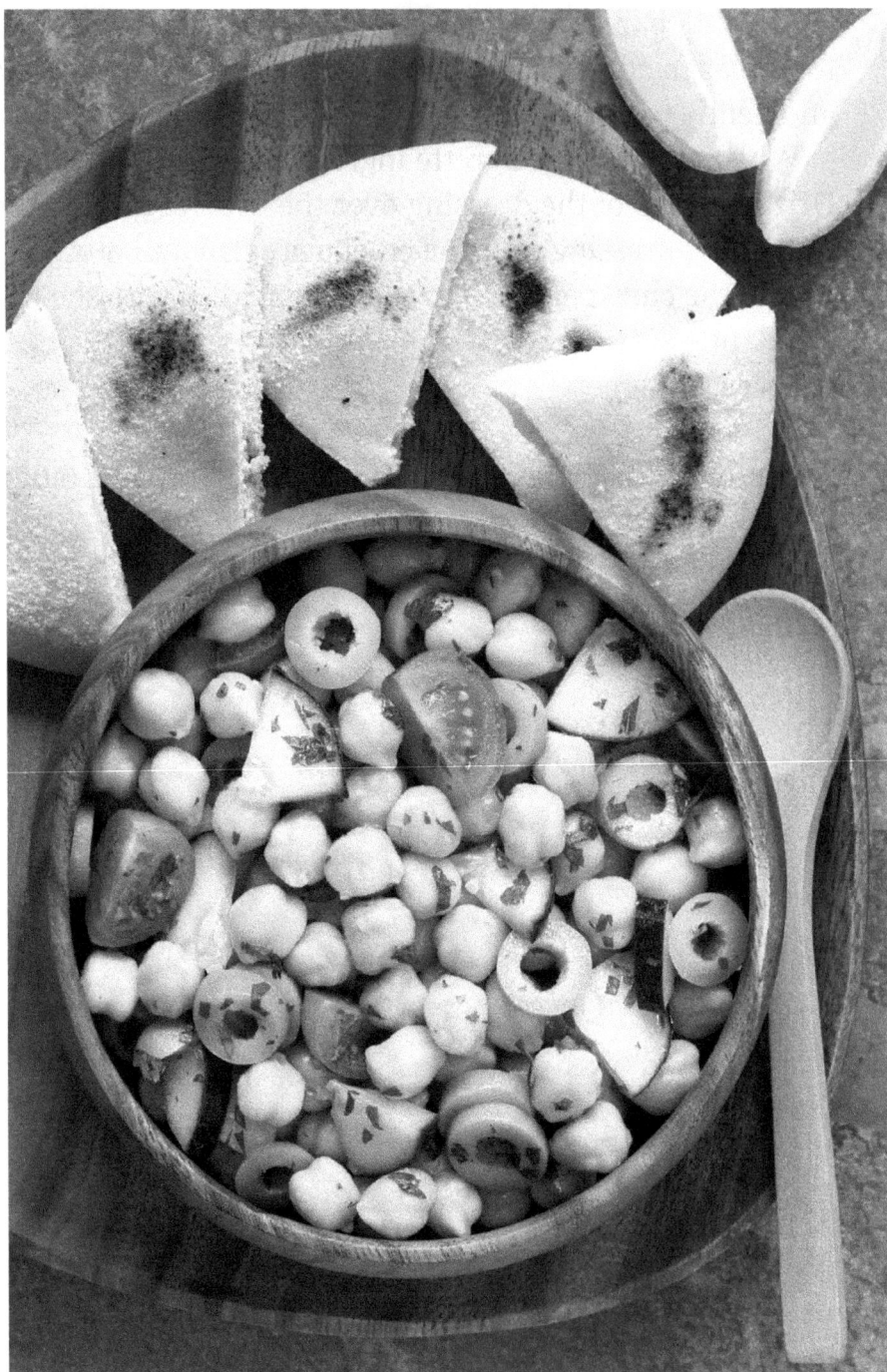

Turkey And Quinoa Stuffed Peppers

Servings: 6
Cooking Time: 55 Minutes

Ingredients:
- 3 large red bell peppers
- 2 tsp chopped fresh rosemary
- 2 tbsp chopped fresh parsley
- 3 tbsp chopped pecans, toasted
- ¼ cup extra virgin olive oil
- ½ cup chicken stock
- ½ lb. fully cooked smoked turkey sausage, diced
- ½ tsp salt
- 2 cups water
- 1 cup uncooked quinoa

Directions:
1. On high fire, place a large saucepan and add salt, water and quinoa. Bring to a boil.
2. Once boiling, reduce fire to a simmer, cover and cook until all water is absorbed around 15 minutes.
3. Uncover quinoa, turn off fire and let it stand for another 5 minutes. 4. Add rosemary, parsley, pecans, olive oil, chicken stock and turkey sausage into pan of quinoa. Mix well.
5. Slice peppers lengthwise in half and discard membranes and seeds. In another boiling pot of water, add peppers, boil for 5 minutes, drain and discard water.
6. Grease a 13 x 9 baking dish and preheat oven to 3500F.
7. Place boiled bell pepper onto prepared baking dish, evenly fill with the quinoa mixture and pop into oven.

8. Bake for 15 minutes.

Nutrition Info: Calories per Serving: 255.6; Carbs: 21.6g; Protein: 14.4g; Fat: 12.4g

Pastitsio An Italian Dish

Servings: 8
Cooking Time: 30 Minutes

Ingredients:
- 2 tbsp chopped fresh flat leaf parsley
- ¾ cup shredded mozzarella cheese
- 1 3oz package of fat free cream cheese
- ½ cup 1/3 less fat cream cheese
- 1 can 14.5-oz of diced tomatoes, drained
- 2 cups fat free milk
- 1 tbsp all-purpose flour
- ¾ tsp kosher salt
- 5 garlic cloves, minced
- 1 ½ cups chopped onion
- 1 tbsp olive oil
- 1 lb. ground sirloin
- Cooking spray
- 8 oz penne, cooked and drained

Directions:
1. On medium high fire, place a big nonstick saucepan and for five minutes sauté beef. Keep on stirring to break up the pieces of ground meat. Once cooked, remove from pan and drain fat.
2. Using same pan, heat oil and fry onions until soft around four minutes while occasionally stirring.
3. Add garlic and continue cooking for another minute while constantly stirring.
4. Stir in beef and flour, cook for another minute. Mix constantly.

5. Add the fat free cream cheese, less fat cream cheese, tomatoes and milk. Cook until mixture is smooth and heated. Toss in pasta and mix well.

6. Transfer pasta into a greased rectangular glass dish and top with
mozzarella. Cook in a preheated broiler for four minutes. Remove from broiler and garnish with parsley before serving.

Nutrition Info: Calories per Serving: 263; Carbs: 17.8g; Protein: 24.1g; Fat: 10.6g

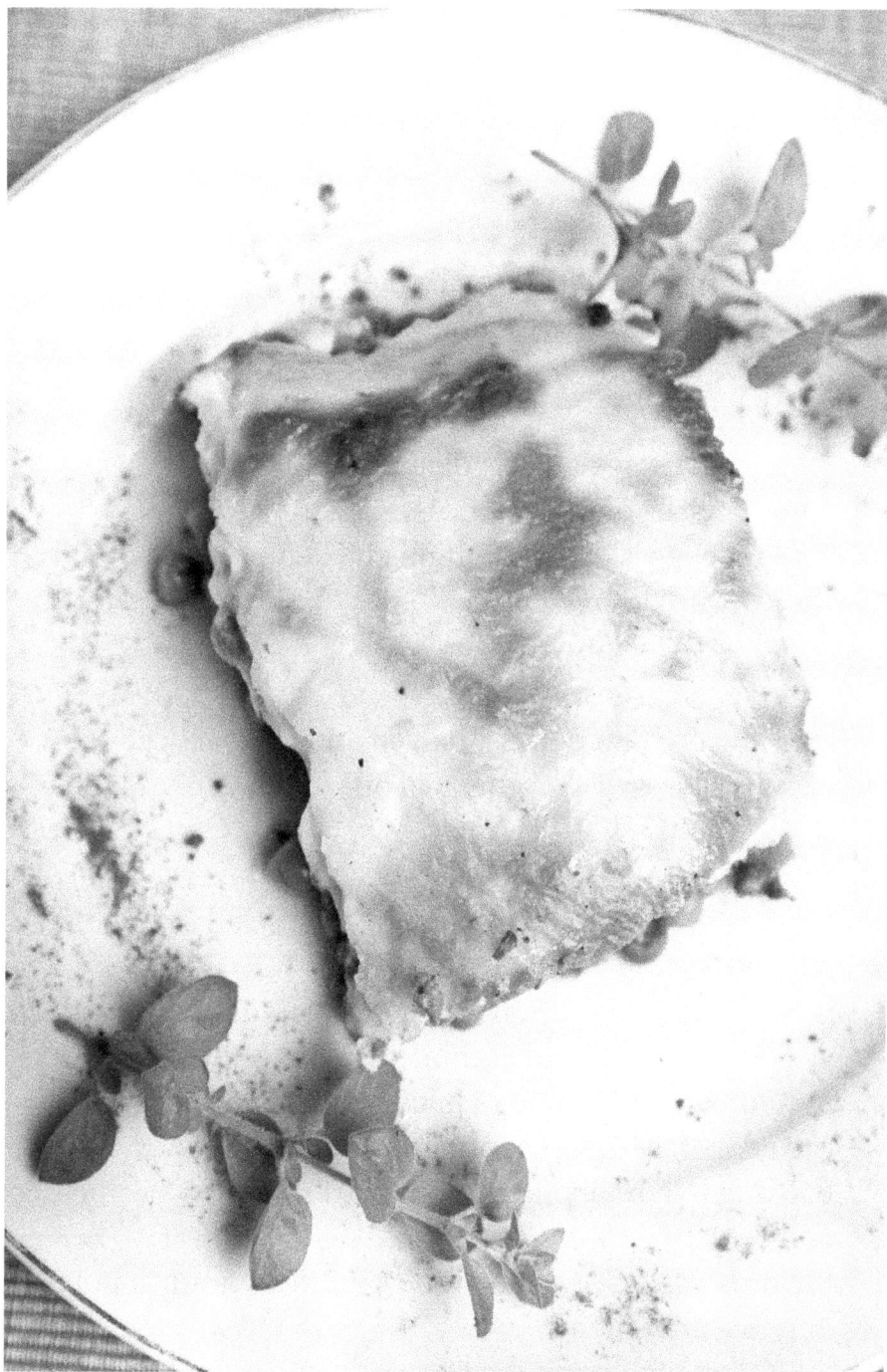

Rice And Chickpea Stew

Servings: 6
Cooking Time: 60 Minutes

Ingredients:
- ½ cup chopped fresh cilantro
- ¼ tsp freshly ground pepper
- ¼ tsp salt
- 2/3 cup brown basmati rice
- 3 cups peeled and diced sweet potato
- 2 15-oz cans chickpeas, rinsed
- 4 cups reduced-sodium chicken broth
- 1 cup orange juice
- 2 tsp ground coriander
- 2 tsp ground cumin
- 3 medium onions, halved and thinly sliced
- 1 tbsp extra virgin olive oil

Directions:
1. On medium fire, place a large nonstick fry pan and heat oil.
2. Sauté onions for 8 minutes or until soft and translucent.
3. Add coriander and cumin, sauté for half a minute.
4. Add broth and orange juice.
5. Add salt, rice, sweet potato, and chickpeas.
6. Bring to a boil, once boiling lower fire to a simmer, cover and cook.
7. Stir occasionally, cook for 45 minutes or until potatoes and rice are tender.
8. Season with pepper.

9. Stew will be thick, if you want a less thick soup, just add water and adjust salt and pepper to taste.
10. To serve, garnish with cilantro.

Nutrition Info: Calories per serving: 332; Protein: 13.01g; Carbs: 55.5g; Fat: 7.5g

Mediterranean Diet Pasta With Mussels

Servings: 4
Cooking Time: 20 Minutes

Ingredients:
- 1 tbsp finely grated lemon zest
- ¼ cup chopped fresh parsley
- Freshly ground pepper to taste
- ¼ tsp salt
- Big pinch of crushed red pepper
- ¾ cup dry white wine
- 2 lbs. mussels, cleaned
- Big pinch of saffron threads soaked in 2 tbsp of water
- 1 can of 15 oz crushed tomatoes with basil
- 2 large cloves garlic, chopped
- ¼ cup extra virgin olive oil
- 8 oz whole wheat linguine or spaghetti

Directions:
1. Cook your pasta following the package label, drain and set aside while covering it to keep it warm.
2. On medium heat, place a large pan and heat oil. Sauté for two to three minutes the garlic and add the saffron plus liquid and the crushed tomatoes. Let it simmer for five minutes.
3. On high heat and in a different pot, boil the wine and mussels for four to six minutes or until it opens. Then transfer the mussels into a clean bowl while disposing of the unopened ones.

4. Then, with a sieve strain the mussel soup into the tomato sauce, add the red pepper and continue for a minute to simmer the sauce. Lastly, season with pepper and salt.
5. Then transfer half of the sauce into the pasta bowl and toss to mix. Then ladle the pasta into 4 medium sized serving bowls, top with mussels, remaining sauce, lemon zest and parsley in that order before serving.

Nutrition Info: Calories per Serving: 402; Carbs: 26.0g; Protein: 35.0g; Fat: 17.5g

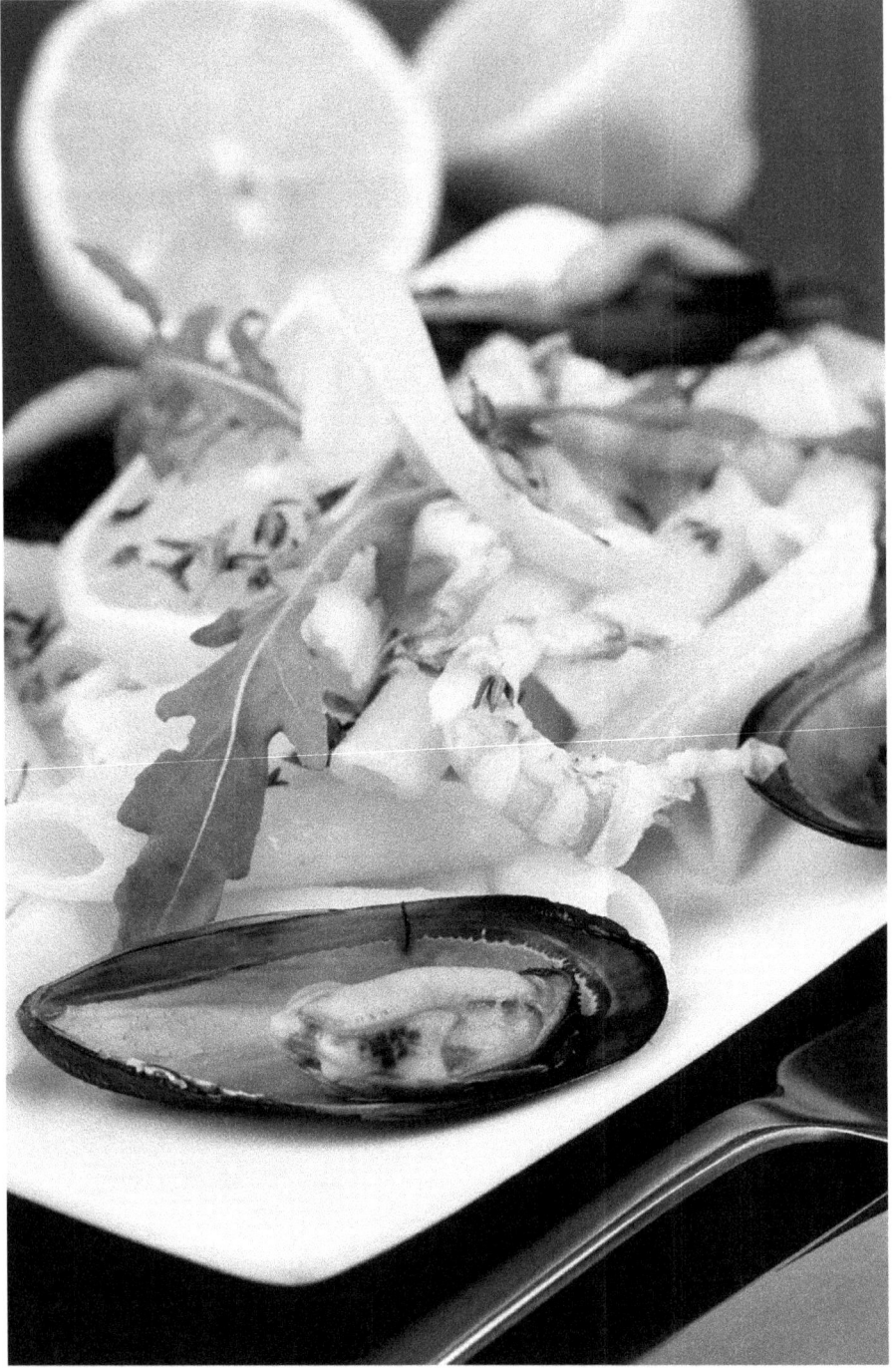

Brussels Sprouts 'n White Bean Medley

Servings: 4
Cooking Time: 15 Minutes

Ingredients:
- 1 tsp salt
- 2 tbsp olive oil
- 3 cans white beans, drained and rinsed
- 3 medium onions, peeled and sliced
- 3 tbsp lemon juice
- 4 ½ cups Brussels sprouts, cleaned and sliced in half
- 6 garlic cloves, smashed, peeled, and minced
- Pepper to taste

Directions:
1. Place a saucepan on medium high fire and heat for 2 minutes.
2. Add oil and heat for a minute.
3. Sauté garlic and onions for 3 minutes.
4. Stir in Brussels Sprouts and sauté for 5 minutes.
5. Stir in white beans and sauté for 5 minutes.
6. Season with pepper and salt.

Nutrition Info: Calories per serving: 371; Protein: 21.4g; Carbs: 57.8g; Fat: 8.1g

Sun-dried Tomatoes And Chickpeas

Servings: 6
Cooking Time: 22 Minutes

Ingredients:
- 1 red bell pepper
- 1/2 cup parsley, chopped
- 1/4 cup red wine vinegar
- 2 14.5-ounce cans chickpeas, drained and rinsed
- 2 cloves garlic, chopped
- 2 cups water
- 2 tablespoons extra-virgin olive oil
- 4 sun-dried tomatoes
- Salt to taste

Directions:
1. Lengthwise, slice bell pepper in half. Place on baking sheet with skin side up. Broil on top rack for 5 minutes until skin is blistered.
2. In a brown paper bag, place the charred bell pepper halves. Fold bag and leave in there for 10 minutes. Remove pepper and peel off skin. Slice into thin strips.
3. Meanwhile, microwave 2 cups of water to boiling. Add the sun-dried tomatoes and leave in to reconstitute for 10 minutes. Drain and slice into thin strips.
4. Whisk well olive oil, garlic, and red wine vinegar.
5. Mix in parsley, sun-dried tomato, bell pepper, and chickpeas. 6. Season with salt to taste and serve.

Nutrition Info: Calories per serving: 195; Protein: 8.0g; Carbs: 26.0g; Fat: 7.0g 645.

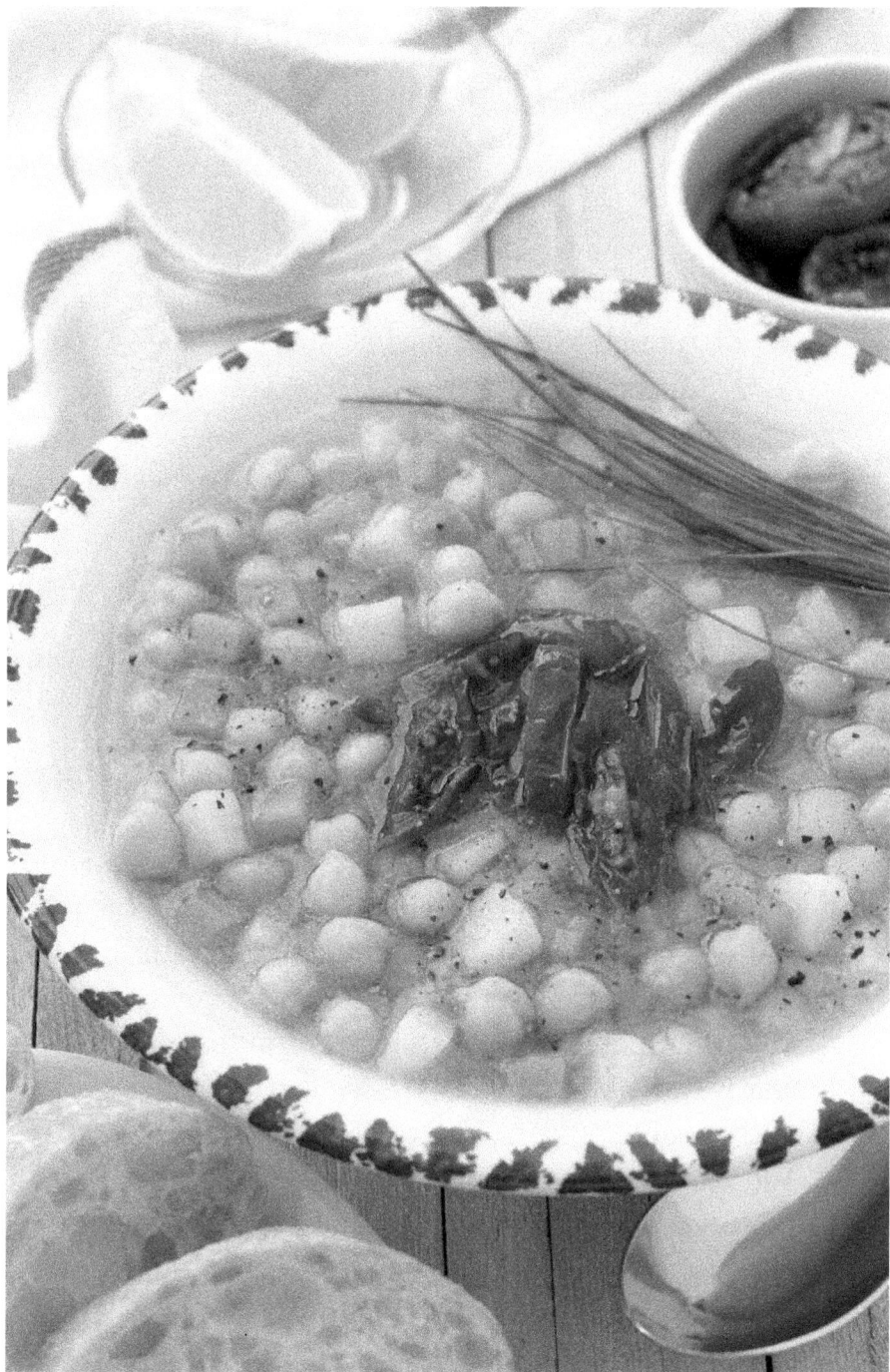

Puttanesca Style Bucatini

Servings: 4
Cooking Time: 40 Minutes

Ingredients:
- 1 tbsp capers, rinsed
- 1 tsp coarsely chopped fresh oregano
- 1 tsp finely chopped garlic
- 1/8 tsp salt
- 12-oz bucatini pasta
- 2 cups coarsely chopped canned no-salt-added whole peeled tomatoes with their juice
- 3 tbsp extra virgin olive oil, divided
- 4 anchovy fillets, chopped
- 8 black Kalamata olives, pitted and sliced into slivers

Directions:
1. Cook bucatini pasta according to package directions. Drain, keep warm, and set aside.
2. On medium fire, place a large nonstick saucepan and heat 2 tbsp oil.
3. Sauté anchovies until it starts to disintegrate.
4. Add garlic and sauté for 15 seconds.
5. Add tomatoes, sauté for 15 to 20 minutes or until no longer watery. Season with 1/8 tsp salt.
6. Add oregano, capers, and olives.
7. Add pasta, sautéing until heated through.
8. To serve, drizzle pasta with remaining olive oil and enjoy.

Nutrition Info: Calories per Serving: 207.4; Carbs: 31g; Protein: 5.1g; Fat: 7g

Garlic Avocado-pesto And Zucchini Pasta

Servings: 2
Cooking Time: 0 Minutes

Ingredients:
- salt and pepper to taste
- 1 tbsp pine nuts
- 1 tbsp cashew nuts
- 1 lemon juice
- 4 cloves garlic, minced
- 1 small ripe avocado
- 2 cups zucchini, spiral
- 2 tbsp olive oil
- 2 tbsp grated Pecorino Cheese
- ½ cup packed fresh basil leaves

Directions:
1. In a food processor grind pine nuts and cashew nuts to a fine powder.
2. Add basil leaves, cheese, olive oil, ripe avocado, garlic, lemon juice, salt and pepper to taste and process until you have a smooth mixture.
3. Arrange zucchini pasta on two plates and top evenly with the Avocado pesto mixture.
4. Serve and enjoy.

Nutrition Info: Calories per Serving: 353; Carbs: 17.0g; Protein: 5.5g; Fat: 31.9g

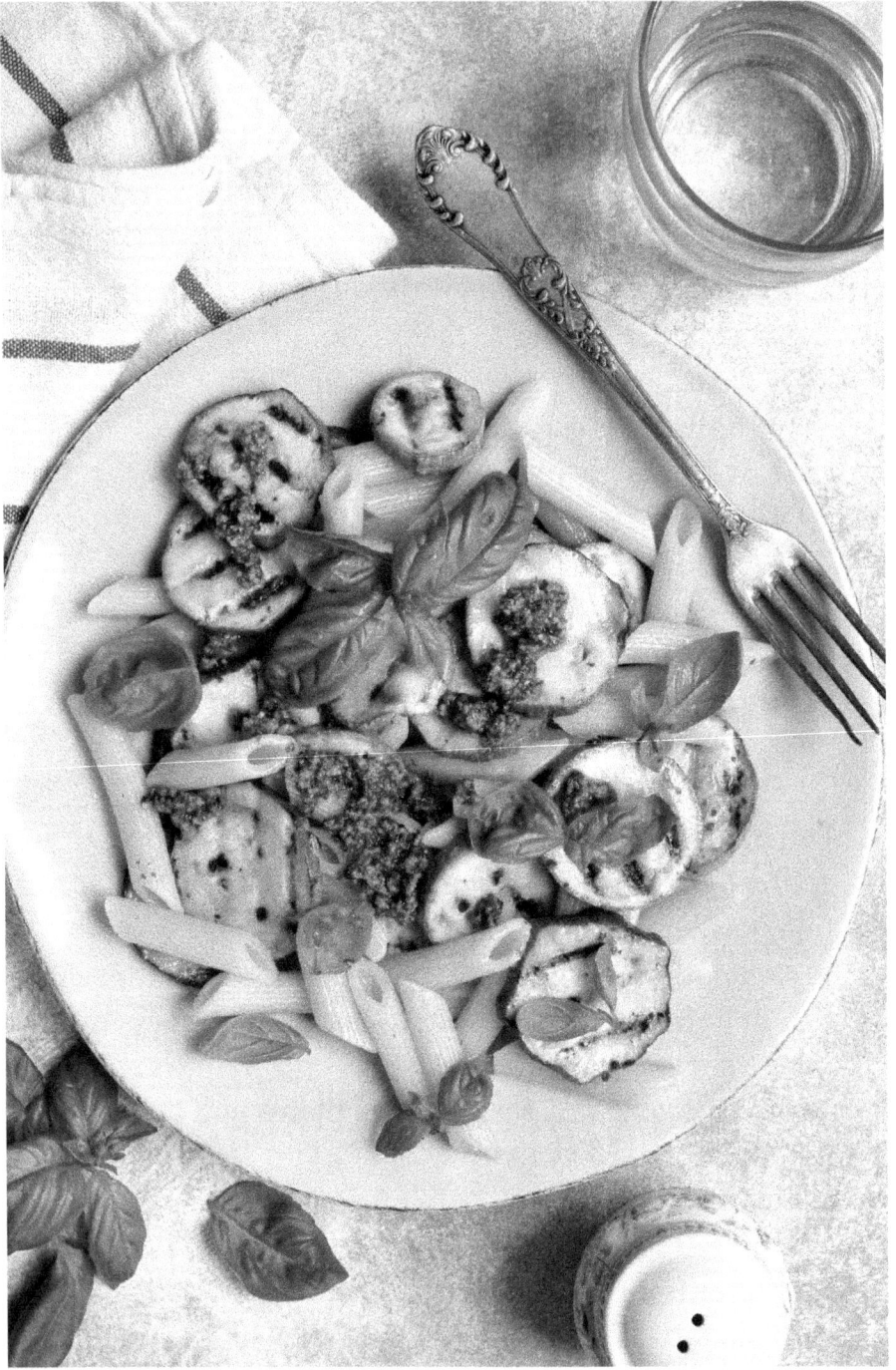

Mushroom Chickpea Marsala

Servings: 4
Cooking Time: 20 Minutes

Ingredients:
- 2 tbsp olive oil
- 8 oz. baby portobello mushrooms, sliced
- 2 garlic cloves, minced
- 1 cup dry Marsala wine
- 2 tbsp lemon juice, or to taste
- 1 tsp rubbed sage
- 1/2 tsp black pepper
- 1/4 tsp salt
- 2 tbsp chopped fresh parsley
- 1-14 oz. can or 1 3/4 cups cooked chickpeas, rinsed and drained

Directions:
1. On medium fire, place a large saucepan and heat oil.
2. Add mushrooms, cover and cook for 5 minutes.
3. Stir in garlic and cook for 2 minutes.
4. Add wine, lemon juice, sage, salt and pepper. Deglaze pot.
5. Simmer for 10 minutes while covered.
6. Add chickpeas and mix well. Cook for 3 minutes.
7. Remove pot from fire and stir in parsley.
8. Serve and enjoy.

Nutrition Info: Calories per serving: 159; Protein: 6.1g; Carbs: 16.8g; Fat: 8.5g

---

Creamy Alfredo Fettuccine

Servings: 4
Cooking Time: 25 Minutes

Ingredients:

- Grated parmesan cheese
- ½ cup freshly grated parmesan cheese
- 1/8 tsp freshly ground black pepper
- ½ tsp salt
- 1 cup whipping cream
- 2 tbsp butter
- 8 oz dried fettuccine, cooked and drained

Directions:
1. On medium high fire, place a big fry pan and heat butter.
2. Add pepper, salt and cream and gently boil for three to five minutes.
3. Once thickened, turn off fire and quickly stir in ½ cup of parmesan cheese. Toss in pasta, mix well.
4. Top with another batch of parmesan cheese and serve.

Nutrition Info: Calories per Serving: 202; Carbs: 21.1g; Protein: 7.9g; Fat: 10.2g

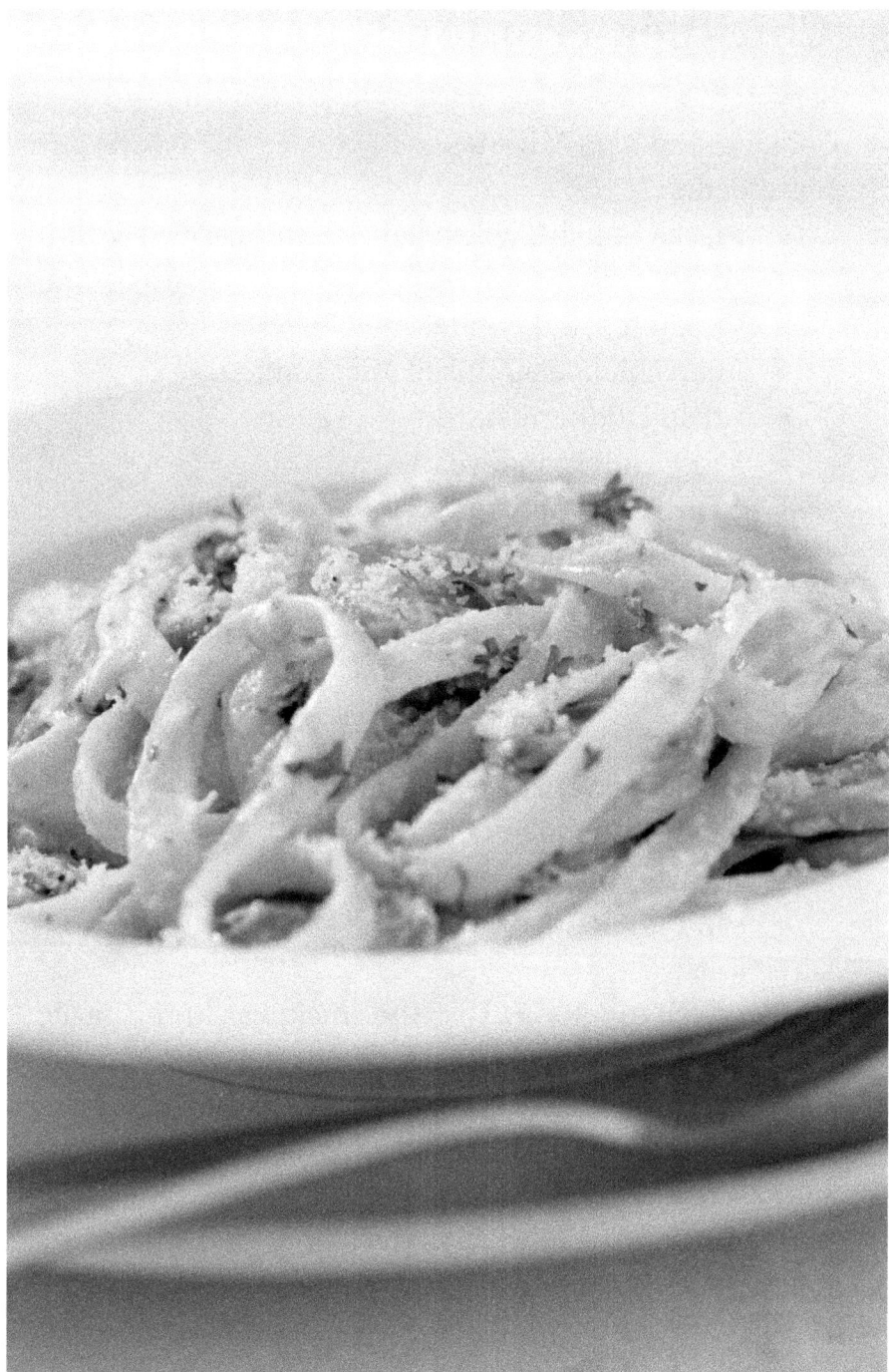

Chickpea-crouton Kale Caesar Salad

Servings: 4

Cooking Time: 35 Minutes

Ingredients:

- 1 large bunch Tuscan kale, stem removed & thinly sliced
- ½ cup toasted pepitas
- 1 cup chickpeas, rinsed and drained
- 1 tbsp Dijon mustard
- 1 tbsp nutritional yeast
- 2 tbsp olive oil
- salt and pepper, to taste
- ½ cup silken tofu
- 2 tablespoons olive oil
- 1 lemon, zested and juiced
- 1 clove garlic
- 2 teaspoons capers, drained
- 2 tablespoons nutritional yeast
- 1 teaspoon Dijon mustard
- salt and pepper, to taste

Directions:

1. Heat oven to 350oF. Toss the chickpeas in the garlic, Dijon, nutritional yeast, olive oil, and salt and pepper. Roast for 30-35 minutes, until browned and crispy.

2. In a blender, add all dressing ingredients. Puree until smooth and creamy.

3. In a large salad bowl, toss the kale with dressing to taste, massaging lightly to tenderize the kale.

4. Top with the chickpea croutons, pepitas, and enjoy!

Nutrition Info: Calories per serving: 327; Protein: 11.9g; Carbs: 20.3g; Fat: 23.8g

Lemon Asparagus Risotto

Servings: 5
Cooking Time: 6 Minutes

Ingredients:
- 1 tablespoons olive oil
- 1 shallot, chopped
- 1 clove of garlic, minced
- 1 ½ cup Arborio rice
- 1/3 cup white wine
- 3 cups vegetable broth
- 1 teaspoon lemon zest
- 2 teaspoon thyme leaves
- Salt and pepper to taste
- 1 bunch asparagus spears, trimmed
- 1 tablespoons butter
- 2 tablespoons parmesan cheese, grated

Directions:
1. Heat olive oil in a pot for 2 minutes.
2. Sauté the shallot and garlic until fragrant, around 2 minutes.
3. Add the Arborio rice and stir for 2 minutes before adding the white wine.
4. Pour in the vegetable broth. Season with salt and pepper to taste.
5. Stir in the lemon zest and thyme leaves.
6. Cover and cook on medium fire for 15 minutes.
7. Stir in the asparagus spears and allow to simmer for 3 minutes.
8. Add the butter and sprinkle with parmesan cheese.

9. Turn off fire and let it sit covered for 10 minutes.

Nutrition Info: Calories per serving: 179; Carbohydrates: 21.4g; Protein:5.7g; Fat: 12.9g

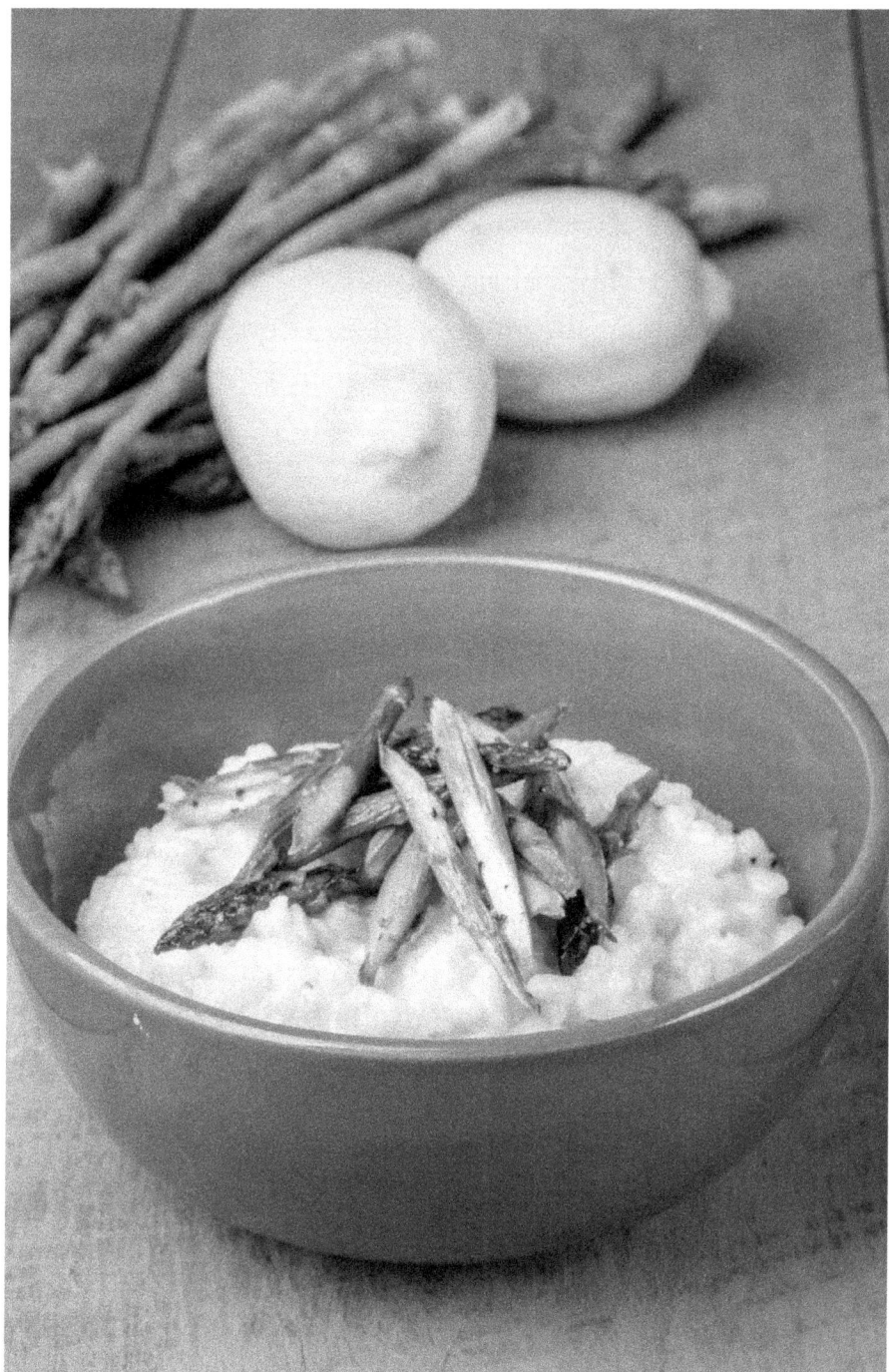

Seafood Paella With Couscous

Servings: 4
Cooking Time: 15 Minutes

Ingredients:
- ½ cup whole wheat couscous
- 4 oz small shrimp, peeled and deveined
- 4 oz bay scallops, tough muscle removed
- ¼ cup vegetable broth
- 1 cup freshly diced tomatoes and juice
- Pinch of crumbled saffron threads
- ¼ tsp freshly ground pepper
- ¼ tsp salt
- ½ tsp fennel seed
- ½ tsp dried thyme
- 1 clove garlic, minced
- 1 medium onion, chopped
- 2 tsp extra virgin olive oil

Directions:
1. Put on medium fire a large saucepan and add oil. Stir in the onion and sauté for three minutes before adding: saffron, pepper, salt, fennel seed, thyme, and garlic. Continue to sauté for another minute.
2. Then add the broth and tomatoes and let boil. Once boiling, reduce the fire, cover and continue to cook for another 2 minutes.
3. Add the scallops and increase fire to medium and stir occasionally and cook for two minutes. Add the shrimp and wait for two minutes more before adding the couscous.

Then remove from fire, cover and set aside for five minutes before carefully mixing.

Nutrition Info: Calories per Serving: 117; Carbs: 11.7g; Protein: 11.5g; Fat: 3.1g

Greek Farro Salad

Servings: 4
Cooking Time: 15 Minutes

Ingredients:
- ½ teaspoon fine-grain sea salt
- 1 cup farro, rinsed
- 1 tablespoon olive oil
- 2 garlic cloves, pressed or minced
- ½ small red onion, chopped and then rinsed under water to mellow the flavor
- 1 avocado, sliced into strips
- 1 cucumber, sliced into thin rounds
- 15 pitted Kalamata olives, sliced into rounds
- 1-pint cherry tomatoes, sliced into rounds
- 2 cups cooked chickpeas (or one 14-ounce can, rinsed and drained) 5 ounces mixed greens
- Lemon wedges
- ⅛ teaspoon salt
- 1 ¼ cups plain Greek yogurt
- 1 ½ tablespoon lightly packed fresh dill, roughly chopped
- 1 ½ tablespoon lightly packed fresh mint, torn into pieces
- 1 tablespoon lemon juice (about ½ lemon)
- 1 tablespoon olive oil

Directions:
1. In a blender, blend and puree all herbed yogurt ingredients and set aside.

---

2. Then cook the farro by placing in a pot filled halfway with water. Bring to a boil, reduce fire to a simmer and cook for 15 minutes or until farro is tender. Drain well. Mix in salt, garlic, and olive oil and fluff to coat.

3. Evenly divide the cooled farro into 4 bowls. Evenly divide the salad ingredients on the 4 farro bowl. Top with ¼ of the yogurt dressing.

4. Serve and enjoy.

Nutrition Info: Calories per serving: 428; Protein: 17.7g; Carbs: 47.6g; Fat: 24.5g

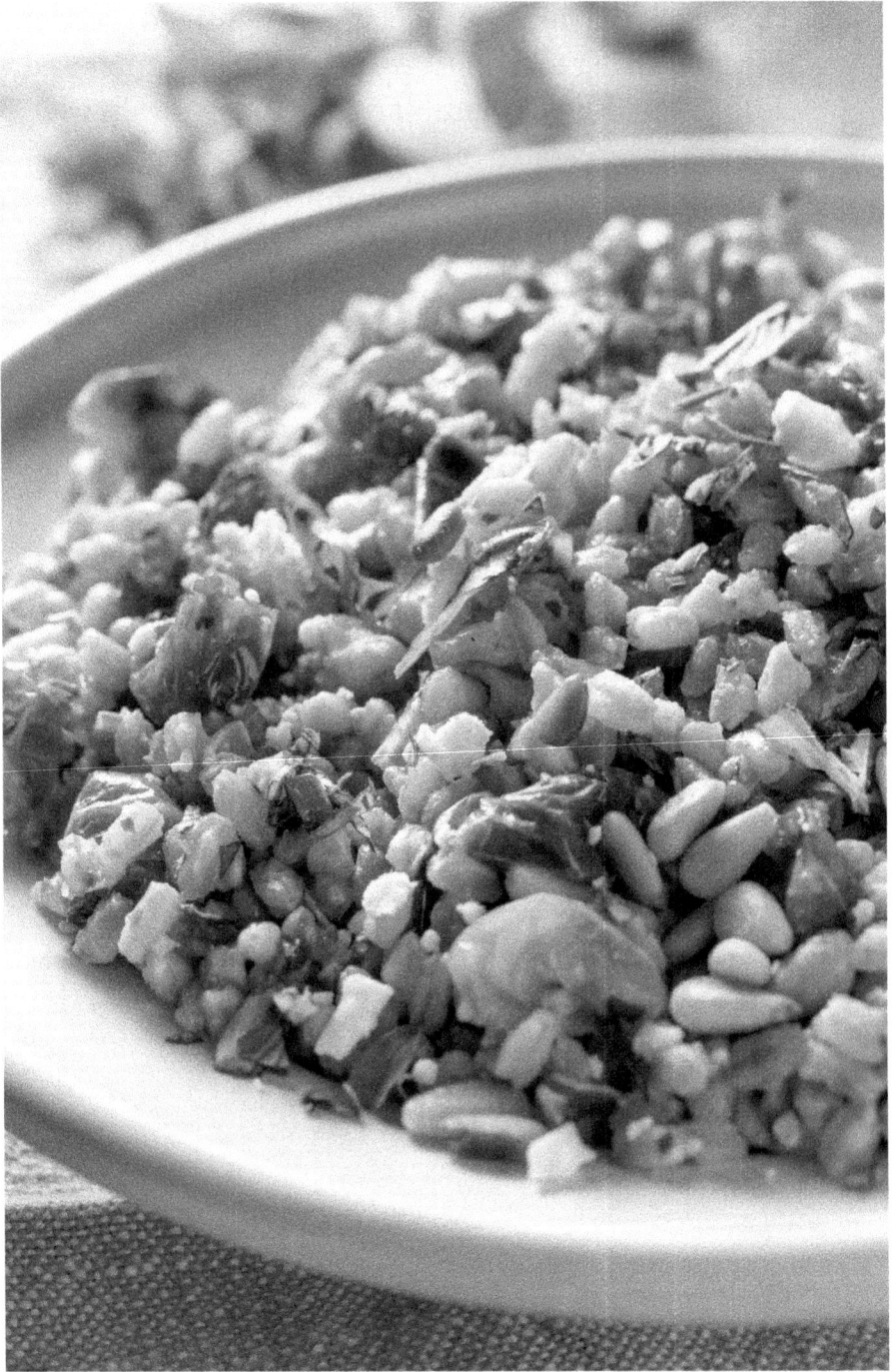

Exotic Chickpea Tagine

Servings: 4
Cooking Time: 45 Minutes

Ingredients:
- 4 tsp sliced toasted almonds
- 1 cup whole wheat couscous, cooked according to manufacturer's instructions
- Freshly squeezed juice of ½ lemon, plus additional to taste
- 1 19-oz can chickpeas, drained and rinsed
- ½ cup water
- ¼ cup packed dried apricots, sliced
- 1 medium zucchini, quartered and cut into ½-inch chunks
- 4 plum tomatoes, cored and chopped
- ¼ tsp turmeric
- 1 whole cinnamon stick
- 1 tsp ground cumin
- 2 tsp honey, plus additional to taste
- ½ tsp harissa paste plus additional to taste
- 3 quarter-sized pieces of peeled fresh ginger
- 2 garlic cloves, roughly chopped
- 2 small carrots, sliced lengthwise, then cut into ½-inch thick slices 1 ½ cups cubed, peeled butternut squash
- ½ tsp salt plus additional to taste
- 1 red onion, quartered and thickly sliced
- 1 ½ tbsp extra virgin olive oil

Directions:

1. On medium low fire, place a heavy and large pot. Heat oil and sauté onions and salt until onions are soft and translucent.

2. Add carrots and sauté for another 5 minutes. Add ginger, garlic and butternut squash. Sauté for 5 minutes and lower fire to medium.

3. Add turmeric, cinnamon stick, cumin, honey and harissa. Sauté for a minute or until fragrant. Stir in apricots, zucchini and tomatoes. Add water and bring to a boil. Once boiling, lower fire to a simmer, cover and cook for 20 minutes or until vegetables are tender.

4. Stir in lemon juice and chickpeas. Increase fire to medium and continue cooking dish uncovered for 5 to 10 minutes or until sauce has thickened.

5. Season dish to taste. Adjust seasoning like lemon, honey and harissa if needed.

6. Serve tagine over couscous and garnished with sliced almonds.

Nutrition Info: Calories per serving: 345; Protein: 13.2g; Carbs: 54.1g; Fat: 10.0g

Amazingly Good Parsley Tabbouleh

Servings: 4
Cooking Time: 15 Minutes

Ingredients:
- ¼ cup chopped fresh mint
- ¼ cup lemon juice
- ¼ tsp salt
- ½ cup bulgur
- ½ tsp minced garlic
- 1 cup water
- 1 small cucumber, peeled, seeded and diced
- 2 cups finely chopped flat-leaf parsley
- 2 tbsp extra virgin olive oil
- 2 tomatoes, diced
- 4 scallions, thinly sliced
- Pepper to taste

Directions:
1. Cook bulgur according to package instructions. Drain and set aside to cool for at least 15 minutes.
2. In a small bowl, mix pepper, salt, garlic, oil, and lemon juice.
3. Transfer bulgur into a large salad bowl and mix in scallions, cucumber, tomatoes, mint, and parsley.
4. Pour in dressing and toss well to coat.
5. Place bowl in ref until chilled before serving.

Nutrition Info: Calories per Serving: 134.8; Carbs: 13g; Protein: 7.2g; Fat: 6g

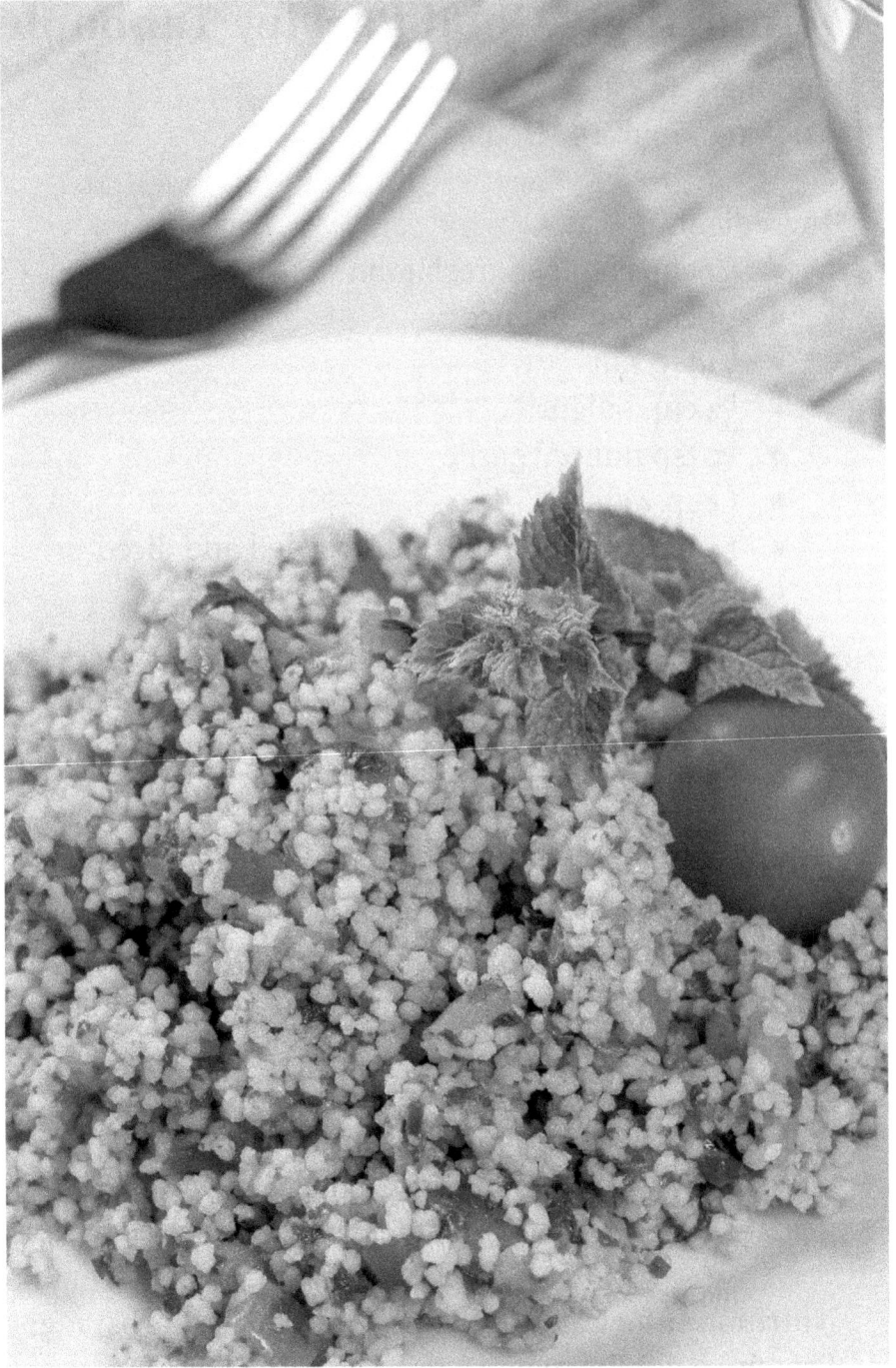

Zucchini And Brown Rice

Servings: 1 Cup
Cooking Time: 50 Minutes

Ingredients:
- 2 TB. extra-virgin olive oil
- 2 large zucchini, diced
- 1 (16-oz.) can artichoke hearts, rinsed and drained
- 1 TB. fresh dill
- 1 tsp. ground black pepper
- 1 tsp. salt
- 4 cups chicken or vegetable broth
- 2 cups basmati brown rice

Directions:
1. In a large, 3-quart pot over medium heat, heat extra-virgin olive oil. Add zucchini, and cook for 3 minutes.
2. Add artichoke hearts, and cook for 2 minutes.
3. Add dill, black pepper, salt, and chicken broth, and bring to a simmer. Stir in basmati brown rice, cover, reduce heat to low, and cook for 40 minutes.
4. Remove from heat, uncover, fluff with a fork, cover, and let sit for another 15 minutes. Serve with Greek yogurt.

Perfect Herb Rice

Servings: 4
Cooking Time: 4 Minutes

Ingredients:
- 1 cup brown rice, rinsed
- 1 tbsp olive oil
- 1 1/2 cups water
- 1/2 cup fresh mix herbs, chopped
- 1 tsp salt

Directions:
1. Add all ingredients into the inner pot of instant pot and stir well.
2. Seal pot with lid and cook on high for 4 minutes.
3. Once done, allow to release pressure naturally for 10 minutes then release remaining using quick release. Remove lid.
4. Stir well and serve.

Nutrition Info: Calories 264 Fat 9.9 g Carbohydrates 36.7 g Sugar 0.4 g Protein 7.3 g Cholesterol 0 mg

Fiber Packed Chicken Rice

Servings: 6
Cooking Time: 16 Minutes

Ingredients:

- 1 lb chicken breast, skinless, boneless, and cut into chunks
- 14.5 oz can cannellini beans
- 4 cups chicken broth
- 2 cups wild rice
- 1 tbsp Italian seasoning
- 1 small onion, chopped
- 1 tbsp garlic, chopped
- 1 tbsp olive oil
- Pepper
- Salt

Directions:

1. Add oil into the inner pot of instant pot and set the pot on sauté mode.
2. Add garlic and onion and sauté for 2 minutes.
3. Add chicken and cook for 2 minutes.
4. Add remaining ingredients and stir well.
5. Seal pot with lid and cook on high for 12 minutes.
6. Once done, release pressure using quick release. Remove lid.
7. Stir well and serve.

Nutrition Info: Calories 399 Fat 6.4 g Carbohydrates 53.4 g Sugar 3 g Protein 31.6 g Cholesterol 50 mg

Baked Parmesan And Eggplant Pasta

Servings: 8
Cooking Time: 50 Minutes

Ingredients:
- ½ tsp dried basil
- ½ cup grated Parmesan cheese, divided
- 8-oz mozzarella cheese, shredded and divided
- 6 cups spaghetti sauce
- 2 cups Italian seasoned breadcrumbs
- ½ lb. ground beef
- 6 cups eggplant, spiralized
- 1 tbsp olive oil

Directions:
1. Grease a 9x13 baking dish and preheat oven to 3500F.
2. On medium high fire, place a nonstick large saucepan and heat oil. Sauté ground beef until cooked around 8 minutes. Pour in spaghetti sauce and cook until heated through.
3. Scoop out two cups of spaghetti meat sauce and set aside.
4. Add eggplant spirals in saucepan and mix well.
5. Scoop out half of eggplant spaghetti into baking dish, top with half of mozzarella cheese and cover with breadcrumbs. Top again with the remaining spaghetti, mozzarella and Parmesan cheese.
6. Pop into oven and bake until tops are golden brown around 35 minutes.
7. Remove from oven and evenly slice into 8 pieces.

8. Serve and enjoy while warm.

Nutrition Info: Calories per Serving: 297; Carbs: 26.6g; Protein: 22.9g; Fat: 11.1g

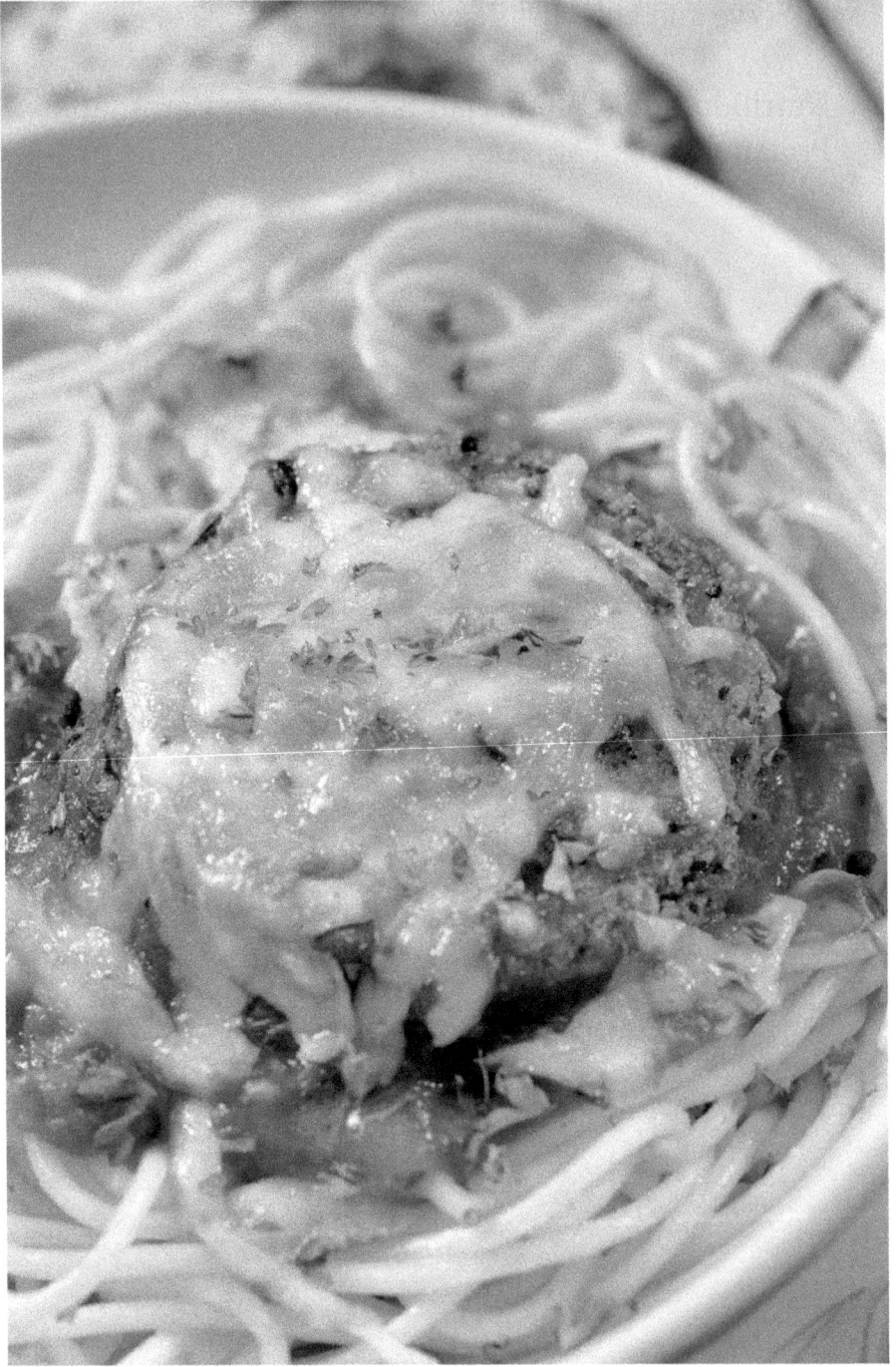

Greek Couscous Salad And Herbed Lamb Chops

Servings: 4
Cooking Time: 30 Minutes

Ingredients:
- ¼ tsp salt
- ½ cup crumbled feta
- ½ cup whole wheat couscous
- 1 cup water
- 1 medium cucumber, peeled and chopped
- 1 tbsp finely chopped fresh parsley
- 1 tbsp minced garlic
- 2 ½ lbs. lamb loin chops, trimmed of fat
- 2 medium tomatoes, chopped
- 2 tbsp finely chopped fresh dill
- 2 tsp extra virgin olive oil
- 3 tbsp lemon juice

Directions:
1. On medium saucepan, add water and bring to a boil.
2. Ibn a small bowl, mix salt, parsley, and garlic. Rub onto lamb chops.
3. On medium high fire, place a large nonstick saucepan and heat oil.
4. Pan fry lamb chops for 5 minutes per side or to desired doneness. Once done, turn off fire and keep warm.
5. On saucepan of boiling water, add couscous. Once boiling, lower fire to a simmer, cover and cook for two minutes.

6. After two minutes, turn off fire, cover and let it stand for 5 minutes.

7. Fluff couscous with a fork and place into a medium bowl.

8. Add dill, lemon juice, feta, cucumber, and tomatoes in bowl of couscous and toss well to combine.

9. Serve lamb chops with a side of couscous and enjoy.

Nutrition Info: Calories per Serving: 524.1; Carbs: 12.3g; Protein: 61.8g; Fat: 25.3g

Fresh Herbs And Clams Linguine

Servings: 4
Cooking Time: 10 Minutes

Ingredients:
- ½ tsp freshly ground black pepper
- ¾ tsp salt
- 2 tbsp butter
- 1.5 lbs. littleneck clams
- ½ cup white wine
- 4 garlic cloves, sliced
- ¼ tsp crushed red pepper
- 2 cups vertically sliced red onion
- 2 tbsp olive oil
- 2 tsp grated lemon zest
- 1 tbsp chopped fresh oregano
- 1/3 cup parsley leaves
- 8-oz linguine, cooked and drained

Directions:
1. Chop finely lemon rind, oregano and parsley. Set aside.
2. On medium high fire, place a nonstick fry pan with olive oil and fry for four minutes garlic, red pepper and onion.
3. Add clams and wine and cook until shells have opened, around five minutes. Throw any unopened clam.
4. Transfer mixture into a large serving bowl. Add pepper, salt, butter and pasta. Toss to mix well. Serve with parsley garnish.

Nutrition Info: Calories per Serving: 507; Carbs: 53.9g; Protein: 34.2g; Fat: 16.8g

Garbanzo And Lentil Soup

Servings: 8
Cooking Time: 90 Minutes

Ingredients:

- 1 14.5-oz can petite diced tomatoes, undrained
- 2 15-oz cans Garbanzo beans, rinsed and drained
- 1 cup lentils
- 6 cups vegetable broth
- ¼ tsp ground cayenne pepper
- ½ tsp ground cumin
- 1 tsp turmeric
- 1 tsp garam masala
- 1 tsp minced garlic
- 2 tsp grated fresh ginger
- 1 cup diced carrots
- 1 cup chopped celery
- 2 onions, chopped

Directions:
1. On medium high fire, place a heavy bottomed large pot and grease with cooking spray.
2. Add onions and sauté until tender, around three to four minutes.
3. Add celery and carrots. Cook for another five minutes.
4. Add cayenne pepper, cumin, turmeric, ginger, garam masala and garlic, cook for half a minute.
5. Add diced tomatoes, garbanzo beans, lentils and vegetable broth. Bring to a boil.
6. Once boiling, slow fire to a simmer and cook while covered for 90 minutes. Occasionally stir soup.

7. If you want a thicker and creamier soup, you can puree ½ of the pot's content and mix in.

8. Once lentils are soft, turn off fire and serve.

Nutrition Info: Calories per serving: 196; Protein: 10.1g; Carbs: 33.3g; Fat: 3.6g

Pasta And Tuna Salad

Servings: 4
Cooking Time: 12 Minutes

Ingredients:
- ¼ cup mayonnaise
- ¼ cup sliced carrots
- ½ cup chopped zucchini
- 2 cups whole wheat macaroni, uncooked
- 1/3 cup diced onion
- 2 5-oz cans low-sodium tuna, water pack

Directions:
1. In a pot of boiling water, cook macaroni according to manufacturer's instructions.
2. Drain macaroni, run under cold tap water until cool and set aside.
3. Drain and discard tuna liquid.
4. Place tuna in a salad bowl.
5. Add zucchini, carrots, drained macaroni and onion. Toss to mix.
6. Add mayonnaise and mix well.
7. Serve and enjoy.

Nutrition Info: Calories per Serving: 168.2; Carbs: 24.6g; Protein: 5.3g; Fat: 5.4g

Quinoa Buffalo Bites

Servings: 4
Cooking Time: 15 Minutes

Ingredients:
2 cups cooked quinoa
1 cup shredded mozzarella
1/2 cup buffalo sauce
1/4 cup +1 Tbsp flour
1 egg
1/4 cup chopped cilantro
1 small onion, diced

Directions:
1. Preheat oven to 3500F.
2. Mix all ingredients in large bowl.
3. Press mixture into greased mini muffin tins.
4. Bake for approximately 15 minutes or until bites are golden.
5. Enjoy on its own or with blue cheese or ranch dip.

Nutrition Info: Calories per serving: 212; Carbs: 30.6g; Protein: 15.9g; Fat: 3.0g

Feta On Tomato-black Bean

Servings: 8
Cooking Time: 0 Minutes

Ingredients:
- 1/2 red onion, sliced
- 1/4 cup crumbled feta cheese
- 1/4 cup fresh dill, chopped
- 2 14.5-ounce cans black beans, drained and rinsed
- 2 tablespoons extra-virgin olive oil
- 4 Roma or plum tomatoes, diced
- Juice of 1 lemon
- Salt to taste

Directions:
1. Except for feta, mix well all ingredients in a salad bowl.
2. Sprinkle with feta.
3. Serve and enjoy.

Nutrition Info: Calories per serving: 121; Protein: 6.0g;
Carbs: 15.0g; Fat: 5.0g 665. Black